Neck and Back Pain

A self-help guide

D0279924

A How To **Self-Help Guide**

Neck and Back Pain

A practical guide to getting on with your life

Dr Chris Jenner

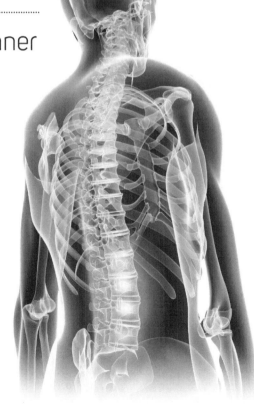

howtobooks

Published by How To Books Ltd
Spring Hill House, Spring Hill Road
Begbroke, Oxford OX5 1RX
Tel: (01865) 375794. Fax: (01865) 379162
info@howtobooks.co.uk
www.howtobooks.co.uk

How To Books greatly reduce the carbon footprint of their books by sourcing
their typesetting and printing in the UK.

All rights reserved. No part of this work may be reproduced or stored in an
information retrieval system (other than for purposes of review) without the
express permission of the publisher in writing.

The right of Christopher Jenner to be identified as author of this work has been
asserted by him in accordance with the Copyright, Designs and Patents Act
1988.

© 2011 Christopher Jenner

British Library Cataloguing in Publication Data
A catalogue record for this book is available from the British Library

ISBN 978 0 84528 468 8

Produced for How To Books by Deer Park Productions, Tavistock
Typeset by PDQ Typesetting Ltd, Newcastle-under-Lyme, Staffs.
Printed and bound in Great Britain by MPG Books Group, Bodmin, Cornwall

NOTE: The material contained in this book is set out in good faith for general
guidance and no liability can be accepted for loss or expense incurred as a result
of relying in particular circumstances or statements made in the book. The laws
and regulations are complex and liable to change, and readers should check the
current position with the relevant authorities before making personal arrangements.

Contents

Contents

Part Two: Living with Neck and Back Pain

Part Three: Managing and Treating Neck and Back Pain

Preface

When we think about back pain, for many of us the image which comes to mind is of an elderly relative or neighbour struggling tentatively to rise from a chair and declaring 'Ooh, me back!' Back and neck pain, however, are not just the preserves of the elderly and they are certainly no laughing matter.

It is estimated that somewhere around 80% of adults will experience back pain at some point in their lives, and as much as two-thirds of the population will suffer the effects of neck pain. This makes these two particular afflictions some of the most costly in terms of healthcare and time lost from work. More significantly though, they are responsible for the suffering of literally millions of people and are two major causes of disability.

Despite being areas of the body that many take for granted, the neck and back are two of the most vulnerable to accident and injury, not to mention the natural process of ageing and the wear and tear inflicted as we go about our daily activities. The complex construction of the spine, as well as the huge number of muscles, tendons and ligaments, all mean that there is enormous potential for something to go wrong and, when it does, the effects on our lives can be devastating.

For most people, neck or back pain, which strikes without warning, and sometimes without any apparent reason, is frightening. Both the severity of the pain and the restrictions to mobility which are often experienced make it easy to imagine that some terrible injury or disease must be at the root of the problem. As symptoms continue for days, weeks and months, sometimes without much response to over-the-counter or prescription medications and sometimes without doctors having been able to determine which of the bewildering array of neck or back disorders is responsible for the distress, it begins to look increasingly possible that quality of life has been lost forever, or even that the sufferer's days may be numbered.

The good news about neck and back pain is that the overwhelming majority of cases involve nothing serious, and most are only short-lived. The potential for acute neck or back pain to develop into a chronic condition, however, can be high, and what many people are surprised to learn is just how much control they themselves have over whether this happens. Their decisions, their choices and their instinctive behaviours can all help to dictate the ultimate impact of their condition on the quality of their lives and the extent of their suffering.

With such a wide range of potential causes, symptoms which could point to an assortment of different underlying problems and a variety of treatments which affect different patients in different ways, cases involving neck and back pain are undoubtedly complex. Their ability to impact considerably, not only on physical well-being, but on emotional and psychological health too, only adds to the problem. The prognosis, however, is far from hopeless, and with a multi-disciplinary approach to neck and back pain, thousands of people have been able to eradicate pain, restore levels of mobility and improve their quality of life immensely.

In this book, you will learn about the different types of neck and back pain and get to grips with some of the often confusing terms that medical professionals use when talking about these types of conditions. You will discover the symptoms and the causes, as well as learning what to expect when your case is being diagnosed and the vast range of treatment options that may be recommended. As this book has been written exclusively with the sufferer in mind, it makes no assumption that the reader has any prior medical knowledge and so the information is set out in simple, straightforward language which is accessible to all.

Because living with neck and back pain can have such far-reaching implications in terms of sufferers' home, family, social and working lives, however, this book does not just stop at considering the essential medical facts. Just as importantly, it provides vital information concerning the effects of neck and back pain on everyday lives and advice on what sufferers can do to minimise these.

Living free of pain and experiencing a good quality of life IS possible, even in the case of chronic neck and back conditions, but understanding is the key to making the very best decisions and choices. It is my sincere hope that by the time you reach the end of this book, you too will feel empowered to join the ranks of those who have learned to live happily, comfortably and successfully despite their conditions.

Dr Christopher Jenner MB BS, FCRA
London Pain Clinic

Part One

Understanding Neck and Back Pain

Different Types of
Neck and Back Pain

The Oxford English Dictionary defines pain as 'physical suffering or discomfort caused by illness or injury', but many would argue that this falls short of describing the real experience in that it fails to take account of the emotional suffering which typically accompanies the physical sensations. In its definition, therefore, the International Association for the Study of Pain describes pain as 'an unpleasant sensory and emotional experience associated with actual or potential tissue damage or described in terms of such damage', a definition which clearly gets one step closer to acknowledging the potential of pain to have a wider impact on our lives.

With the notable exception of the pain of contractions during childbirth, which is the only positive and constructive pain there is, pain is always a sign that something is not right. When a part of our body is hurt or when we become sick, the nerves from the affected area of the body send messages to the brain to let us know that all is not well. In this way, although probably only in this way, pain can be thought of as a positive thing, because it acts as a warning system and prompts us to take some kind of action to protect our bodies.

Neck and back pain are two notoriously complex types of pain but, like pain in other parts of the body, they can still be classified in a number of different ways. Not only is it helpful to understand these in order to make sense of a doctor's diagnosis, but also to help you understand the treatment which is prescribed. As different types of pain respond differently to certain types of treatment, determining what type of pain you are experiencing allows your medical care specialist to ensure that the chosen course of action is the most appropriate and effective to deal with your particular case.

Classifying pain according to time

One of the main ways of classifying pain is time-related and most readers will have heard of the terms acute pain, chronic pain and recurring pain. These, however, are frequently misunderstood and are often believed to be connected with the intensity of pain rather than the period of time over which the sensations are felt or the regularity of painful episodes. Here, therefore, is a quick guide as to what each term actually relates to in a medical sense.

Acute pain

Although the term 'acute pain' tends to suggest to many people pain which is sharp or intense, when doctors use it they are actually referring to pain which has been present for a relatively short period of time, typically less than three months. Acute pain might indeed be felt as sharp, but it could also present as a dull, nagging ache. Whatever the sensation, however, it is usually a constant pain which varies in terms of its intensity. It might, for example, feel worse when you move in a particular way, but then settle down to a 'normal' level when you adopt a different posture or cease the activity which caused the flare-up.

Acute pain very often occurs as the result of an injury, due to inflammation or because of a disease and it normally comes on fairly suddenly. In the case of acute neck and back pain, both the immediacy of the discomfort and the fact that the pain can spread to other areas of the body can make it feel particularly distressing to the sufferer, but most of the time neck pain in particular will resolve itself within 7–10 days with rest, ice and over-the-counter pain relievers.

In the case of an accident, of course, professional medical advice should be sought immediately to ensure that the full extent of any injuries are assessed and that proper treatment is prescribed. If the cause of the pain is unknown, however, or if initial treatment after an accident or injury does not resolve the problem, then patients are advised to wait no more than a few weeks before receiving a thorough evaluation from a medical professional.

Chronic pain

Again, the term 'chronic pain' tends to be thought of as severe pain but, when doctors diagnose pain as being chronic, what they mean is that it has been experienced continuously for a period of longer than three months. The reason why the three-month timescale is significant in the definitions of acute and chronic pain is because this is the period in which the body would normally heal itself. If you were to experience acute pain from inflammation as the result of taking up a new sport, for instance, the pain might very well go away of its own accord as the affected area healed naturally, especially if the activity was discontinued. However, if the sensations were to continue for longer than three months even after you stopped the activity, then it might suggest an ongoing problem such as damage incurred by a previous injury or a condition such as arthritis or osteoporosis.

Another example might be waking up in the morning with a sore, stiff neck. If the cause was nothing more than sleeping awkwardly, then even if it took a week or two for the symptoms to subside, the body would recover naturally within a relatively short space of time. If your car had been rear-ended in a road accident some time before the onset of the pain and stiffness, however, and the pain continued for longer than three months, then there is a strong likelihood of underlying damage which might require treatment and could respond extremely well to a comprehensive pain management programme.

In terms of its intensity, chronic pain can range from being mild to severe and, where chronic back pain in particular is concerned, it is usually described as being a deep ache or a burning pain which often travels down the legs or into other parts of the body, such as the buttocks. In many cases, sensations of tingling, 'pins and needles' or numbness are also experienced alongside the pain itself and this range of symptoms might continue at a similar level for months, years or even a lifetime without appropriate treatment.

Of course, the very fact that chronic pain goes on for such a long time means that it can have quite a severe impact on the sufferer's quality of life; sleep might be badly affected, daily chores might suffer or it might become difficult, or even impossible, to continue with the same type of work. In addition, both the pain itself, as well as the current and potential future impact on daily life, can very easily lead to anxiety and depression.

Recurring pain

The third type of time-related pain that you are likely to come across is recurring pain which, as the name suggests, is pain which comes and goes. Those who suffer from recurring, or recurrent pain, experience repeated episodes of pain interspersed with periods during which their symptoms disappear entirely.

One of the big problems with recurring pain is that it can sometimes take a while before the sufferer recognises that there is a pattern to their experience, albeit a fairly spasmodic one. Often, those who suffer from recurring pain simply put it down to being 'one of those things', or assume that their symptoms are linked with things like the weather, when actually there could be an underlying problem which requires treatment.

Although recurring pain is not entirely relentless like chronic pain, in some ways it can be equally as distressing, if not more so, because the sufferer cannot enjoy the periods of remission but instead lives in constant fear of the next episode. Especially if the pain that they normally suffer is extreme or the length of time that it generally lasts is prolonged, then their feelings of dread can turn to total preoccupation and problems with anxiety can result. In addition, the fact that the pain keeps coming back tends to suggest to the sufferer some grave underlying cause or even a terminal disease. In nearly all cases, however, the pain is no indicator of a life-threatening illness and it can either be cured totally or managed and treated so that the sufferer experiences considerable and sometimes life-changing relief.

In many cases involving recurrent back pain, it can be difficult for doctors to identify a precise cause. There might be no specific injury to explain the presence of the symptoms and there might be no condition affecting the muscles, nerves, joints or ligaments which account for it either. Even in cases where there has been a previous injury, why the pain comes and goes at certain times might still remain a mystery. As you will discover in the course of reading this book, however, there are certain things which may trigger repeated episodes of pain such as poor posture, compensating for painful areas of the body, limiting your range of movement or even becoming inactive. Stress too can become a factor, as those who live in fear of their next painful episode can experience muscle tension which itself can lead to flare-ups.

Classifying pain according to source

Aside from classifying pain in terms of the length of time during which it has been experienced or how regularly it is present, another way of doing so is according to its source. Broadly speaking, there are three main sources of pain: the musculoskeletal system, the nerves and the internal organs or viscera. As many who have experienced lengthy bouts of pain will know, however, pain which originates from one source can frequently spread to other areas of the body too.

Musculoskeletal pain

Musculoskeletal pain is probably the type which is most familiar to the majority of people and it originates from tissues such as skin, muscle, joints, bones and ligaments. This type of pain activates specific receptors in the body relating to such things as heat, cold, vibration, stretch, inflammation or oxygen starvation and sends messages to the spinal cord and the brain to alert them to the presence of potentially damaging stimuli. Cuts or sprains which cause disruption to the body's tissues and subsequent inflammation, anything which causes muscles to become overstretched or muscle cramps, for example, could be the cause of musculoskeletal pain, which is typically felt as being sharp and localised. Another characteristic of this type of pain is that touching or moving the sensitive area is likely to make the sensation feel worse or, if the sensation has died down, to cause it to start up again.

Musculoskeletal pain can loosely be divided up into that which affects the soft tissues of the body and that which affects the bones. Soft tissue pain is extremely common and can be caused not only by a variety of injuries and illnesses, but also by certain behaviours such as guarding an already injured area. Muscles, tendons and ligaments can all be susceptible to damage, including tearing and stretching, and you do not need to be a sports enthusiast to experience damage to these areas. Whether you are at home, at work or anywhere else, a trip, a fall or lifting something awkwardly can all lead to an injury which causes inflammation and soft tissue pain, and of course repetitive activities can play havoc with muscles and tendons as well as nerves.

In cases where an injury has been sustained, musculoskeletal pain can become worse due to the body's natural tendency to protect itself by tensing the muscles. Not only can the constant contraction of the muscles itself cause pain to muscles, tendons, fascia and nerves, but muscles which are contracted for any length of time can effectively become stuck and unable to relax, and this can lead to the development of the tender points and trigger points (sensitive areas which cause localised pain or refer pain to other parts of the body) which are characteristic of illnesses such as fibromyalgia and myofascial pain syndrome. In addition, the circulation to the affected area becomes restricted so that it does not receive the amount of oxygen that it needs to keep it functioning normally. Even in cases where we have experienced no form of physical injury but have become very stressed, this same inclination to tense the body can have precisely the same results.

Perhaps one of the less well-known sources of musculoskeletal pain is that which comes from the fascia or connective tissue of the body. Despite being nothing more than a very thin, clear membrane, the fascia plays an important role in supporting and dividing the muscles, organs and nerves, and even the blood vessels and bones throughout our entire bodies, and if it suffers any damage, such as through dehydration, it can not only affect the way that different areas of the body interact with one another, but even our posture.

Musculoskeletal pain does not just originate from the soft tissues of the body, but also from the bones or the joints which connect the bones, and osteoarthritis and rheumatoid arthritis are just two examples of conditions which typically cause this type of pain. Not only can the joints become inflamed and swollen, but eventually they can become so badly damaged that bone is rubbing on bone. Even being overweight can cause joints to become compressed to such an extent that the cartilage is worn away and pain is the result. In other cases, the problem stems from the bone itself, such as is the case when extra areas of bony growth develop and then begin pushing against the soft tissues and interfering with the normal joint function.

Nerve pain

Nerve pain, otherwise known as neuropathic pain, comes from within the nervous system itself, either from the nerves which are found between the tissues and the spinal cord (the peripheral nervous system) or those between the spinal cord and the brain (the central nervous system). Rather than pain receptors being activated, as is the case with musculoskeletal problems, when a nerve becomes trapped or inflamed it becomes electrically unstable and starts firing off signals in an entirely random or inappropriate manner. These signals are interpreted by the brain as what many would describe as lancing, shooting or burning pain, a dull, throbbing ache or feelings of hypersensitivity, such as to touch, vibration and temperature, tingling, numbness or weakness. Even things such as changes in the weather, certain temperatures or physical touch can bring about sensitivity in damaged or injured nerves.

Where nerve damage has occurred as the result of an injury of some kind, such as a serious cut, sometimes what will happen is that the nerves will continue to send off pain signals long after surrounding tissues and other structures have healed. Because the original injury may not be able to be seen in these cases, it can be difficult for doctors to identify the source of the pain, which of course makes it particularly important that patients provide a full account of their medical history to help with diagnosis.

Nerves, like most other parts of the body, do have at least some ability to heal if the damage they have sustained is not too serious, although the timescale in which this happens can sometimes be lengthy. Where the damage is permanent though, patients can be left with constant pain which, for reasons unknown, generally seems to vary from day to day.

Although, in most cases, nerve pain is caused by the pressure of a trapped nerve, nerve inflammation from a torn or slipped disc or, sometimes, nerve infection due to shingles or other viral infections, it can also result from nerve degeneration as a result of multiple sclerosis, a stroke, a brain haemorrhage or oxygen starvation. These latter causes are, however, much rarer.

Visceral pain

Visceral pain occurs in cases where there has been damage or injury to the internal organs of the body such as the heart, liver, kidneys, spleen or womb. The specific pain receptors which are activated are those for stretch, inflammation and oxygen starvation, but typically the pain which is felt is not localised and is often described as being a vague, deep ache which is sometimes cramping or colicky in nature.

Visceral pain is known for its common tendency to refer pain to various areas of the back. Pelvic pain, which originates from the bladder, womb and ovaries, often refers to the lower back, while abdominal pain originating from the liver, kidneys, spleen and bowels, frequently refers to the middle part of the back. Thoracic pain, meanwhile, which stems from the heart and lungs, tends to be referred to the upper back.

Combinations of pain

Pain which originates from one source can lead to pain from other sources, so creating combinations of pain. A good example of this might be if an individual sustained damage to a nerve and then began tensing the surrounding muscles, which there is a natural tendency to do. The muscle tension, as we saw when we looked at musculoskeletal pain, would then begin to create a secondary source of pain. The same might be true if the person were to 'guard' an injury, perhaps by adopting a different gait or posture. By forcing surrounding areas of the body into what are essentially unnatural positions, there is every likelihood that the musculoskeletal system would respond with further pain.

Many chronic pain syndromes in particular are made up of different types of pain which it is important that doctors are able to classify. Only by doing so can medical professionals combine the appropriate medications, treatments and therapies to achieve the very best in terms of pain management.

What is neck pain?

The term 'neck pain' can refer to any sensation of soreness, aching or discomfort in any of the structures of the neck, including the muscles, the nerves, the upper part of the spinal column which extends up the back of the neck to the base of the skull (known as the cervical vertebrae) and the spinal discs which act as a buffer between each of the vertebrae. The pain can range from being mild to severe and it might remain at the same level of intensity or get progressively worse. In addition, it might be acute, chronic or recurring and it can arise due to a whole number of different reasons, although rarely are these very serious in nature.

The pain which is experienced, however, does not necessarily emanate directly from the neck area and is not necessarily confined solely to it. In fact, it can come from the shoulders, jaw, head or upper arms, all of which are near the neck, and it can also spread into the shoulders, upper back, arms, hands, fingers and head. Wherever it starts or spreads to though, neck pain can make movement extremely difficult and can restrict normal daily activities quite severely. If you have ever woken up in the morning with a crick in your neck, you will understand just how painful and awkward it is to drive, for example, and in situations such as this of course, it does not just hurt, but it can be dangerous too.

Like so many parts of our bodies, our necks are typically taken very much for granted. Actually though, because the cervical vertebrae allow our necks and heads so much movement, this makes it an especially vulnerable part of our anatomy, and only when we start to experience problems do we come to appreciate just how extensively it is used. Especially when neck pain is severe or long-lasting, it is considerably more than just 'a pain in the neck' to live with and, alongside making even normal daily life quite a challenge, it can even lead to fatigue, depression and anxiety.

Alongside the more general classifications of pain that we have already looked at, neck pain itself can be divided up into three different types:

- **axial neck pain** is musculoskeletal pain which affects the soft tissues or muscles of the neck, and it is the type of pain which might be experienced in the wake of a whiplash or muscle strain injury, for example;
- **cervical radiculopathy** refers to pain in the neck and arm which is caused by nerve root compression. The symptoms of this type of pain generally include arm pain, numbness or weakness;

■ *myelopathy* occurs when there is pressure on the spinal cord. Myelopathy can cause neck pain, along with weakness or numbness in the arm and/or leg or difficulties in walking.

Although it is quite common for people to think that spinal pain is more common in the older members of society, in fact numerous studies have shown this not to be the case. In terms of neck pain in particular, if anything it is those of working age who appear to be most susceptible and, when you bear in mind that one study showed that one third of those who took part and who suffered from chronic neck pain had previously sustained a whiplash injury, this is perhaps not very surprising. Indeed, whiplash injuries sustained in motor vehicle accidents are generally considered to be the single most common cause of neck pain, which appears to affect roughly the same number of men as women.

What is back pain?

Back pain is one of the most common reasons for adults to visit a doctor and in fact most people will experience some kind of discomfort in the lower, middle or upper back at some point in their lives. The good news though, is that most episodes of back pain are acute rather than chronic (although chronic back pain is still widespread), and that these cases of acute back pain tend to clear up within just one month.

The back is not only a large area of the body, but it is one which is complex in terms of the arrangement of bones, ligaments, muscles, joints and nerves, consisting of:

■ 24 small bones which make up the vertebrae to support the weight of the upper body and act as protection for the spinal cord;
■ the spine's shock-absorbers or intervertebral discs which cushion the bones and allow the spine to bend;
■ ligaments to hold the vertebrae and discs together;
■ tendons to connect muscles to vertebrae;
■ the spinal cord, which carries nerve signals from the brain to the rest of the body;
■ numerous nerves and muscles.

There is, unfortunately, plenty to go wrong. In fact, in the UK, chronic back pain is reported to be the second most common cause of long-term disability after arthritis and the leading cause of long-term work-related absence. In the USA, meanwhile, back pain is believed to be the number one cause of disability in workers under the age of 45.

Of the three main parts of the back, it is the lower back, or the lumbar region, which is responsible for most of the pain and stiffness that individuals experience. This region is made up of five vertebrae which are numbered L1, L2, L3, L4 and L5 from top to bottom, and it is the part of the back which not only supports the entire weight of the upper body, but also any additional weight that you carry or lift. Being under constant pressure then, and especially when you bend, twist or lift, it is most susceptible to damage or injury irrespective of your age.

Like neck pain, back pain too has its own set of classifications, these being specific back pain and non-specific back pain. Specific back pain is that which is associated with damage to the spine or an underlying health condition, while non-specific back pain, rather than being caused by serious damage or disease, is caused by compressed or inflamed nerves, sprains, muscle strains and minor injuries.

Although back pain is no respecter of age or gender, certain individuals are believed to be more at risk of experiencing it than others. As you might expect, those whose work involves heavy labour, lots of lifting or a considerable amount of vibration in the back area are particularly susceptible, but so too are people who spend long periods of time either sitting or standing. People who have allowed themselves to become out of shape can also be more at risk if their abdominal and back muscles have become weak and additional strain is placed on the muscles and joints of the back. Smokers too, are also believed to suffer more from back pain than non-smokers.

Quite worryingly, cases of back pain in the UK and almost all western nations are reported to have doubled during the course of the past 40 years. Some put this down to the fact that people are more willing to report their symptoms to a doctor nowadays than they were previously, but perhaps just as likely is that obesity, depression and stress are also taking their toll on our health. Despite the complex nature of the spine and the back region though, the much greater understanding of the doctors of today means that problems can be diagnosed and treated much more effectively than they were years ago.

2

Know the Symptoms

Pain is the body's way of letting us know that all is not as it should be. Pain is not the only symptom that something is wrong however. Rashes, coughs, sensations such as tingling or weakness and all manner of other signs can all alert us to a problem. Knowing what is 'normal' and what could potentially be a sign of illness or injury, therefore, is important if we are to take the right course of action.

There are those people who would contend that for laypeople to know a little about the symptoms of a condition is a dangerous thing and that it can lead to hypochondria or jumping to the very worst kinds of conclusions. Awareness, however, can literally save lives. Think, for example, about blood poisoning or septicaemia. Anyone who is aware of the significance of that telltale red line making its way inexorably, and often very quickly, along the veins and towards the heart would know that they needed to seek urgent medical attention and that leaving it for a day or two could prove fatal. Similarly, knowing that severe stiffness in the neck is just one of the symptoms of meningitis just might encourage an anxious parent to take action sooner rather than later.

Knowing under what circumstances to seek help and how urgently is not the only reason for understanding a bit about symptoms though, because the awareness of patients can also help doctors to make faster and more accurate diagnoses. You may, for example, experience symptoms which appear insignificant, unrelated or irrelevant, and so not bother to report these to your doctor. Actually though, they could be of great significance and could make the world of difference in terms of diagnosing the problem correctly and prescribing the most appropriate and effective treatment. Being able to identify and describe the absence or presence of certain symptoms can essentially help your doctor to help you.

An awareness of symptoms should, however, never lead you down the road of self-diagnosis. Diagnosing illness in general is often a complex matter which requires years of medical training and experience, and the numerous structures of the neck and back and the many potential causes of neck and back pain mean that particular care needs to be taken when establishing the nature of problems in these areas and prescribing the right kind of treatment. Missing certain signs or dismissing them as irrelevant could not only allow certain conditions or injuries to go unchecked and untreated, but it could also lead you to indulge in activities or behaviours which cause the problem to worsen.

Throughout the remainder of this chapter, I will look at some of the main symptoms associated with neck and back problems, as well as at some of the red flags which might act as a warning to take more urgent action. Do be aware, however, that reading about them is no substitute for seeking proper professional advice and a thorough medical evaluation.

The symptoms of neck pain

Even though most of us will experience at least one episode of neck pain during our lives, the sensations that we feel are likely to vary enormously. For some, it might be nothing more than slight stiffness, whilst for others it could be severe pain or any of a whole range of different feelings which are not limited to the neck itself. Here are some of the main symptoms which characterise problems associated with the neck:

- pain which is felt solely in the neck, from the bottom of the head to the top of the shoulders, or which spreads to the shoulders, upper back or arms;
- pain which is felt just on one side of the neck;
- neck pain which is worse with movement
- stiffness, tenderness or what feels like a knot in the neck which may limit the movement of the head and neck;
- generalised pain in the shoulder or arm;
- sharp pain which shoots down the arm;

- numbness or tingling in the arms, hands or fingers;
- weakness in the hands or arms which may cause you to drop things;
- a burning sensation when the skin of the arm or hand is touched;
- weakness or numbness in the legs or tripping or stumbling when walking;
- headaches which may be mild or severe and which may persist for months;
- dizziness;
- weight loss;
- nausea;
- loss of the ability to control urination or bowel movements.

Although some of these symptoms sound undeniably frightening and, particularly when they are experienced over prolonged periods of time, can have a huge impact on a sufferer's quality of life, in most cases the cause of the problem is not something serious or one which necessitates anything as drastic as surgery. There are, though, certain occasions when neck pain or stiffness and/or certain other symptoms can indicate the need for emergency medical investigation, such as:

- when stiffness in the neck is such that the patient cannot touch the chin to the chest and the stiffness is accompanied by fever, headaches and possibly (although not always) a rash which does not fade under pressure. These are the classic signs of meningitis, a condition which can worsen extremely quickly and can be life-threatening. If these symptoms are present, you should immediately call the local emergency number (999 in the UK or 911 in the USA) or get to a hospital straight away;
- when the ability to control urination or bowel movements is lost. One of the reasons why this can happen is that there is considerable pressure on, or injury to the spinal cord. Again, seek emergency medical attention;
- when the neck pain was caused by a fall, a blow or an injury. In these circumstances, it is vital that your condition is properly assessed in order to detect any damage which may not be immediately obvious. If neck pain is accompanied by the loss of the use of a hand or arm, then again you should call the emergency number or get yourself to a hospital.

If, however, you or somebody that you know is experiencing any of the following symptoms, these should always be checked out by a medical professional:

- neck pain which is accompanied by a fever, chills and weight loss;
- sensation of numbness, tingling or weakness in the arms, hands or legs;
- loss of balance;
- severe headaches;
- dizziness;
- symptoms which persist after one week despite a self-care programme;
- pain which does not respond to regular doses of over-the-counter pain medication;
- swollen glands or a lump in the neck;
- neck pain accompanied by difficulties in breathing or swallowing;
- neck pain which has no obvious cause;
- neck pain which is getting progressively worse over time;
- neck pain which worsens when you lie down or which keeps you awake at night;
- neck pain which goes on for longer than three weeks.

The symptoms of back pain

Back pain is characterised by pain, aching or stiffness in any area of the upper, middle or lower regions of the back. In some cases it might present as a sharp pain which is experienced, for example, after lifting something heavy, whilst in others it might feel like a chronic ache after sitting or standing for long periods of time. Some people experience tightness or pulling, but it could also present as a burning or throbbing sensation.

The pain might be constant or intermittent, it might vary in terms of the level of intensity or remain at the same level and its onset may be sudden or more gradual. Also, it may be more prevalent at different times of the day, such as when the sufferer wakes up in the morning.

As with neck pain, there are certain occasions or symptoms which should act as red flags where back pain is concerned, and you should always seek immediate medical attention if:

- severe pain lasts for more than a few days without any improvement and does not ease after lying down or resting;

- the pain is constant and getting worse;
- the pain is affecting your normal everyday activities;
- the pain makes it difficult for you to bend forwards;
- back pain is accompanied by fever or weight loss;
- back pain is accompanied by numbness, tingling or weakness in the hands or arms;
- there is inflammation or swelling on the back;
- back pain is accompanied by difficulty in passing urine or the loss of bladder or bowel control;
- numbness is experienced in the back or in the area around the genitals, anus or buttocks;
- numbness, weakness or pins and needles are felt in the legs;
- there is a shooting pain down the leg;
- the pain continues down the legs to below the knees;
- the pain travels to the chest or is experienced high up in the back;
- unsteadiness is experienced when standing;
- the pain has resulted from a recent injury or trauma to the back;
- severe lower back pain is accompanied by pain in the abdomen;
- back pain is accompanied by an obvious structural deformity of the spine.

Certain groups of people are also advised to seek medical advice if they experience the onset of back pain, including:

- those who are younger than 20 or older than 55 and who are experiencing their first episode of back pain;
- those who have or have had cancer;
- drug abusers;
- those who have been taking steroids for at least a few months;
- those who have a low immune system as a result of chemotherapy, HIV/AIDS or another medical condition.

With both neck and back pain, it is important to remember that muscle tension caused by stress is only likely to cause the pain to worsen or other types of pain to develop. Rather than being in a constant state of worry about the cause of the pain, therefore, it is always better to seek professional medical advice so that the relevant treatment can be prescribed and started without delay.

Understanding the Causes

Neck and back pain are some of the commonest types of pain to be experienced by adults around the world today, particularly in the West. They can occur as the result of accident, injury, trauma, stress, developmental disorders and a variety of medical conditions, some of which may be inherited.

Understanding the causes of neck and back pain is helpful for two quite separate reasons. Firstly, being aware of those which are within our control can help us to avoid them, and secondly, a greater knowledge can often be very effective in terms of relieving the fear that many people feel when they experience these types of conditions. In this chapter, therefore, we are going to take a look at some of the causes of neck and back pain in an attempt to demystify them. Before we go on to do this, however, let me just take a moment to explain the anatomy of the spine, which will make understanding some of these causes much easier.

The back is made up of three separate regions: the upper, middle and lower regions. The spine, of course, passes through each of these areas, and it too is divided up for medical purposes into three different sections. Starting at the top, these are known as the cervical, thoracic and lumbar spine, and each section is made up of a number of individual bones called vertebrae. The cervical spine or neck has seven vertebrae (numbered C1–C7), the thoracic or middle section of the spine has 12 (numbered T1–T12) and the lumbar or lower section has five (numbered L1–L5). The numbering system that doctors use for the vertebrae always begins from the bone at the top of each section and works down.

Each vertebra has two upward-facing and two downward-facing facet joints to allow them to link with the vertebrae above and below, and these help to give the spine its stability. In between each of these pairs of bones, meanwhile, is one of the spine's shock absorbers or intervertebral discs, which is made up of an inner portion with a consistency similar to gelatine, called the 'nucleus pulposus', and a fibrous outer ring rather like a tyre which is known as the 'annulus fibrosis'.

Individual vertebrae are each made up of several different parts, of which the body of the vertebra is the main part to bear weight, as well as being the place where the intervertebral discs sit. The lamina, meanwhile, helps to form the central spinal canal through which the spinal cord passes, while the spinous process is the bone that you can feel through your skin and the transverse processes, which sit at a 90° angle to the spinous process, provide attachment for the back muscles. In addition, there are 31 pairs of nerve roots which branch off from the spinal cord, numerous fibrous, slightly stretchy ligaments connecting bone to bone, a hugely elaborate system of arteries and veins and, in the neck alone, there are 32 separate muscles. The ligaments and muscles not only help to support the spine, but also to prevent excessive movement which could lead to injury.

With all this complex machinery, clearly there is much that can go wrong with the human neck and back. Even when it is not being subjected to any type of additional stress or trauma, for example, the neck has to support the full weight of the head, which is typically around eight pounds, and on top of this it also has to move the head freely in a variety of directions. In fact, the cervical spine can move the head 90° in a forward direction and the same backwards, 180° from side to side and it can also tilt the head almost 120° down towards each shoulder. That's quite a lot of work!

Bearing in mind all the movement and the stresses and strains that the neck has to put up with, it normally does an exceptionally good job of staying fit and healthy. Having said this though, it is its very flexibility which makes the cervical spine somewhat vulnerable to injury, with the number one cause being the whiplash type injury that so many people suffer as the result of motoring accidents. Of course, when it does suffer trauma, or when it starts to degenerate through wear and tear or because of illness, it is then that neck pain and associated pains and stiffness can become a problem.

The back, meanwhile, has its own fair share of abuse to try and withstand as we go about our everyday activities, and it is typically the minor injuries, muscle strains or pinched nerves that we incur as we do so which account for the vast majority of cases of lower back pain in particular. Poor posture, bending awkwardly, lifting incorrectly, twisting, over-stretching and standing, bending or driving for long periods of time, along with simple things like coughing and sneezing, can all cause pain which might last for days, weeks, months or even years. In some cases, we cannot even remember what it was that we did to set it off.

Of course, these are not the only causes of back pain, however. More serious trips or falls can sometimes cause quite extensive injuries or damage to the back, such as fractures, whilst obesity and pregnancy bring their own pressures to bear, quite literally. Certain types of arthritis, infections, developmental disorders, as well as a host of other causes, including a number of other medical conditions, all conspire to make back pain such a common complaint, and of course as we age, we additionally become more susceptible to the degeneration process.

The causes of neck and back pain that you will find laid out in alphabetical order in the following pages are some of the more common ones, but it is worth pointing out that some are very much more common than others. Although it may be tempting to read through and fear the worst, do try to bear in mind that even in cases where the intensity of the pain feels quite high, the cause is most often relatively minor and the pain itself can be treated and managed very effectively in order to restore your quality of life. As you will see, with the right care, the prognosis for the majority of cases of neck and back pain is actually extremely good!

Accidents and injuries

Whiplash injuries sustained in motoring accidents are responsible for the majority of cases of neck pain, but of course these are not the only kind which can cause injury or damage to the neck. Slips, trips and falls, as well as sudden twisting movements, can all be responsible for sprains and strains which affect the ligaments and the muscles of the neck.

Ligament sprains happen when the ligaments which connect the vertebrae stretch beyond their normal limits and then snap back into place suddenly, leaving them either stretched or torn. This is one of the common characteristics of a whiplash injury and the symptoms usually include pain in the back of the neck which worsens with movement, pain in the sides of the neck and muscle spasms or pain in the upper parts of the shoulders and back. Headaches, which tend to be felt in the back of the head, are also common, as is neck stiffness, and sometimes those with neck sprains also experience a sore throat. Typically, the pain associated with neck sprains does not manifest itself until 24 to 48 hours after the accident which caused them.

Of course, one very common cause of neck problems, and sprains in particular, is sports injuries. While almost any kind of sport could potentially lead to a neck sprain, it is contact sports such as rugby, football, hockey and basketball which present the greatest risk for players.

As well as being responsible for many of the cases of neck pain which are reported to doctors every year, muscle and ligament strains and sprains also account for the majority of incidents of acute back pain. Despite their size and strength, the muscles in the lower back or lumbar region are particularly prone to rips and tears; these muscle strains are most commonly caused by lifting or bending awkwardly, lifting objects which are too heavy or applying sudden force to the muscles before they are ready for activity. Not only does the muscle itself rip, but also the blood vessels within the muscle tissue, which can cause bleeding into the injured area. Often though, it will be several hours before the injury causes sufficient irritation or bleeding to produce pain, which means that sometimes people will continue with their activities unaware of the damage that has been inflicted and may even incur further damage as a result. Only later will they experience the intense pain, swelling and muscle spasms which are typical of muscle strain injuries.

Ligament sprains to the back are also a common cause of back pain and, as is the case with neck sprains, it is the overstretching of the ligaments which causes the problem. Again, bending, twisting and lifting are responsible for most ligament sprains, and those whose sedentary lifestyles have caused weakness in the lower back are most susceptible to these and muscle strains.

Particularly where injury has been caused by a major fall or a motor vehicle accident, it is not uncommon for the accident victim to sustain both muscle strains and ligament sprains. The pain which is experienced as a result of these injuries can be very severe and may last for weeks or even months. In some cases, the area around the site of the injury can become inflamed, causing painful muscle spasms and difficulty in moving, but generally back strains and sprains can be treated effectively to relieve the pain and ensure full recovery. Only in extremely rare cases would surgery be recommended as an appropriate course of treatment with these types of injuries.

The soft tissues in the neck and back are not, of course, the only vulnerable parts of these bodily structures and the injuries sustained as a result of falls, motor vehicle accidents and so on can also include bone fractures. In some cases these may be fairly insignificant and require nothing more than the wearing of a cervical collar, for instance, but in other more serious cases there may be a need for surgery to correct any instability of the spine that the injury may have caused and/or to repair damaged nerves.

Ankylosing spondylitis

Ankylosing spondylitis is a progressive form of inflammatory arthritis which causes the joints and ligaments of the lower part of the spine to become inflamed. The early symptoms present as chronic pain and stiffness in the lower back, or sometimes the whole of the spine, and often there is referred pain to either of the buttocks or the back of the thigh. The pain is generally felt whether at rest or when moving, but in some cases physical activity can help to lessen the pain. The condition, which tends to be inherited, can eventually cause fusion of the spine so that it becomes completely rigid. In addition, it can affect other joints in the body, as well as the eyes, lungs and the heart.

Although it can also occur in women, ankylosing spondylitis tends to affect mostly males between the ages of 16 and 30, but regardless of gender, most patients with the condition have a gene called HLA-B27. Males tend to suffer higher levels of pain than females, as do those who contract the condition before the age of 18, and suffer swelling of the joints in the limbs, especially the knee. Younger sufferers can also experience pain and swelling in the ankles and feet.

Because the body tries to heal itself of the condition by creating new vertical bony outgrowths which can fuse the vertebrae together and make the spine completely inflexible, the earlier it can be treated the better. If treatment is delayed, then fusion can stiffen the rib cage and interfere with the functioning and capacity of the lungs.

Where ankylosing spondylitis becomes severe enough to require surgery to realign the bones, the patient's posture will typically be such that the head is bent forwards so that the chin is almost resting on the chest. Aside from the stooped appearance, there would also be chronic stiffness and a decreased range of motion, and the individual may be experiencing fatigue, loss of appetite and sometimes fever.

Although the precise cause of ankylosing spondylitis is not known and there is also no known cure, it is not a fatal condition and the prognosis is generally good. In many cases, patients have long periods of remission during which they experience few or no symptoms, and those who suffer from the condition can generally expect to lead normal and productive lives. Despite being chronic in nature, ankylosing spondylitis rarely causes severe disability and in most cases the condition can be managed very successfully and without surgery becoming a requirement.

The two main keys to managing the condition are controlling pain and inflammation, and doctors may therefore prescribe anti-inflammatory drugs or corticosteroids to reduce swelling, as well as pain-relieving medications. Exercise too is an important part of treatment and is aimed at strengthening the back and abdominal muscles, as well as restoring flexibility to the spine. Physical therapy and other types of manipulative treatments can also be significant in terms of offering pain relief and increasing mobility, but it is also important for posture to be addressed as part of the treatment regime. As is the case with the treatment of all types of neck and back problems, however, there is no 'one size fits all' treatment package and each individual patient's programme needs to be designed to suit them specifically and adjusted to ensure the most beneficial effects.

Bulging disc

In a normal spine, the intervertebral discs sit in line with the bones themselves and do not protrude at all around the edges. Often as a result of age, however, the jelly-like substance inside the disc begins to press on the outer wall, causing the whole thing to bulge out from between the two vertebrae. In itself, this is not actually a problem and indeed, in many cases, the effects of a bulging disc might not be felt at all. If it starts to press on the nerves of the spine, however, it can become extremely painful, as well as causing symptoms such as numbness and tingling. If the nerve is pinched for a prolonged period of time, it can even cause irreversible damage.

Where age is the most significant factor in causing bulging discs, it is because the outer wall of the disc has lost its elasticity and started to weaken. Age, however, is not the only thing which can be responsible for this condition and, as you might expect, those who are heavier in weight are at greater risk because of the increased pressure on the discs. Taller people are also believed to be more susceptible, as are those whose work involves a great deal of heavy lifting or bending and, according to some studies at least, smokers. Trauma to the spine and some degenerative diseases can also cause intervertebral discs to bulge.

Although it is very common for bulging discs to cause pain in the lower back, often with pain radiating into the legs, they can sometimes occur in the neck area too. Where this is the case and there is pressure on a nerve or it becomes pinched, pain is usually felt in the shoulders and arms, as well as the neck.

Bulging discs, which are quite different from herniated or ruptured discs, are often not picked up until other back or neck problems such as general strains or sprains are investigated. When persistent pain starts to become an issue, therefore, it is important that the source be properly established, as clearly the treatment may vary according to the diagnosis.

In many cases involving bulging discs, the treatment prescribed is likely to include anti-inflammatory medications or cortisone injections, along with medication to relieve the pain. Heat or ice therapy, as well as physical therapy, may also be recommended and normally the patient would be advised to rest and avoid putting any undue strain on the back or neck while the inflammation of the spinal nerve has a chance to die down. Only in cases where the bulging disc becomes herniated and the individual is experiencing severe pain due to nerve compression would surgery ordinarily be deemed to be appropriate.

In most cases, a programme of conservative treatment (i.e. that which does not involve surgery) does much to relieve the pain and discomfort of a bulging disc and, in certain cases, the pain may be completely resolved. Although the bulge never really disappears entirely, there is still enough of the disc sitting between the vertebrae to avoid any further degeneration taking place and, once medication and physical therapy have provided some relief to the affected nerves, re-education in terms of posture and movement can help to ensure that painful episodes are minimised.

Collapsed vertebra

The vertebrae which give much of the structural support to the spine, like other bones in the body, can of course sustain damage as a result of injury or disease. Particularly in cases where trauma to the back is caused by a vertical shock (such as due to a fall from a great height or being catapulted from an ejector seat), and those in which the vertebrae have become considerably weakened as a result of conditions such as osteoporosis, one or more vertebrae can suffer compression fractures and effectively collapse or become crushed.

Compression fractures or collapsed vertebrae occur most commonly in the lower thoracic or upper lumbar region of the spine and usually the damage is to the body of the bone which is at the front. The back of the vertebra, where the spinal cord and nerves are situated, is typically unaffected, which means that the bone takes on a wedge-shaped appearance and causes the spine to curve forwards. Often, patients who suffer compression fractures notice a decrease in their overall height because the spinal column has effectively been shortened.

Patients who suffer from osteoporosis experience a thinning of the bones which can eventually lead to vertebrae collapsing in on themselves and compression fractures to result. Where the vertebrae have become significantly weakened as a result of the condition, it does not necessarily take a serious fall or injury for such a fracture to occur and even going about daily activities can be enough to cause one or more of the bones to collapse.

In some very serious cases of trauma to the spine, not only is the front part of the bone affected, but the body of the vertebra is crushed in all directions. This is known as a burst fracture and is a much more severe type of injury, both because it can result in damage to the nerves and spinal cord which can even cause paralysis and because it causes the spine to become much less stable. Cases involving burst fractures typically require immediate treatment to relieve or prevent any pressure on the spinal cord or the nerves.

The pain associated with collapsed vertebrae is normally severe and patients also often experience severe limitation in their ability to move. There may be some minor swelling, as well as a reduction in sensation to the extremities and, where there is any pinching of the spinal cord, tingling or numbness may be experienced in various parts of the body.

Despite the serious-sounding nature of compression fractures, usually there is no requirement for an operation to fix them. With the help of anti-inflammatory medication, restrictions to activity and the wearing of a brace or cast, the damaged vertebrae will normally heal themselves very successfully within the course of eight to twelve weeks. Medication for pain relief will also be administered during this period as required.

If the pain is chronic, however, and the patient does not respond well to other types of pain management, it may become necessary for either a vertebroplasty or a kyphoplasty to be performed. While the first of these procedures is aimed at stabilising the fracture and involves the injection of medical-grade bone epoxy or glue into the affected vertebrae, the second helps to restore the height or the shape of the bones by using a cement-like substance. A vertebroplasty only involves minimal invasion and so there is usually no requirement for the patient to undergo an overnight stay in hospital, although 24 hours of bed rest is normally recommended. Normal activities can generally be resumed within a couple of days. A kyphoplasty, on the other hand, requires a small incision to be made in the back, a hospital stay and 24 hours of bed rest after returning home. Normal activities can be resumed gradually as they can be tolerated, but lifting is not recommended for at least six weeks after the operation.

Although the prognosis for collapsed vertebrae is normally good, those who have suffered one compression fracture are at greater risk of experiencing more. Learning about prevention, therefore, is important, and especially for sufferers of osteoporosis.

Degenerative or osteoarthritis

Degenerative arthritis is often referred to in the medical profession as spinal arthritis, arthritis of the facet joints, degenerative joint disease, spondylosis or osteoarthritis of the spine. Osteoarthritis, which literally means arthritis of the bone, is not only the most common form of arthritis, but also one of the most frequently disabling, and it is a condition which causes the cartilage which protects and cushions the bones to break down. When this happens, the sufferer generally experiences pain and swelling and, if the ends of the affected bones start to rub together and osteophytes or bone spurs form and become large enough, these too can cause irritation as well as trapped nerves.

Generally, osteoarthritis is a condition which affects people as they age and it is most likely to occur after the age of 45–50. In this age group it is more common in women, but in the under 45s it is more prevalent amongst men. In addition, it occurs more frequently in those who are overweight, as well as in those whose jobs or hobbies put repeated stress on particular joints. Younger people who suffer from osteoarthritis generally do so because of an injury or trauma to a joint, a genetic defect which affects cartilage or a condition which causes the joint to lose its proper formation.

In osteoarthritis of the spine, it is the cartilage between the facet joints, which help to support the weight and control the movement between individual vertebrae, which is affected. Most commonly this occurs in the neck and lower back and, as the cartilage wears away in these areas, the friction between the joints causes pain and the spine begins to stiffen and lose its flexibility. If the nerves are affected, then weakness and pain in the arms or legs can also become a problem.

Most people who suffer from the condition complain that the pain feels worse first thing in the morning, decreases throughout the course of the day and then worsens again later on. Often it becomes more pronounced when the individual engages in movements which twist or stretch the spine, and typically the pain and discomfort in the back is relieved when the sufferer is lying down.

The effects of osteoarthritis can vary greatly from person to person. While some only experience minimal pain and are able to continue with their normal everyday activities with little or no problem, others can become more severely disabled. Because it is an ongoing degenerative condition, however, often its effects are more than just physical. Increasing restrictions to daily activities can sometimes leave individuals feeling helpless or depressed about their condition, causing them to experience emotional or psychological problems and a sense of isolation.

Another reason why osteoarthritis of the spine can be particularly troublesome is that it often goes hand in hand with degenerative disc disease, which means that the sufferer effectively experiences a double whammy of pain. It is believed that the degeneration of the intervertebral discs puts stress on the facet joints which, over time, leads to the wearing of the cartilage.

The prognosis for halting or slowing the progress of osteoarthritis is currently not good, as there is no proven treatment which will achieve this. However, there are some very effective treatments which can help to relieve the pain and inflammation, strengthen the muscles in the back and restore spinal flexibility and, in most cases, the condition will not become debilitating. Treatment programmes might include pain medications and anti-inflammatory drugs, physiotherapy and manipulative treatments and exercises, and patients may also be advised to go on weight loss diets or stop smoking as appropriate.

Only in the severerest cases would surgery be recommended for patients with degenerative arthritis, as the only effective surgical treatment can itself cause further problems. Fusion, which essentially involves 'welding' two or more vertebrae together, works by stopping any movement of the affected joints, but as the condition typically involves bones at various locations along the spine and multilevel fusions are not generally advisable, doctors will often avoid this course of treatment wherever possible and rely on those which are more conservative. One of the problems which can occur as a result of fusion is adjacent segment degeneration, and I will look at this separately a little further on.

Degenerative disc disease

While degenerative arthritis is concerned with the wearing of the cartilage between the facet joints in the spine, degenerative disc disease, as the name suggests, affects the shock-absorbing discs which sit in between the vertebrae. Despite its somewhat frightening-sounding name, it is actually a perfectly normal part of the ageing process and can be found in individuals as young as 25. Not only this, but it is not strictly a degenerative condition and is not even really a disease.

Basically what happens in degenerative disc disease is that both parts of the intervertebral disc begin to dry out. As the dehydration process affects the nucleus pulposus, the jelly-like substance in the centre, the disc shrinks and the space in between the vertebrae becomes narrower. At the same time, the fibrous outer structure of the disc, the annulus fibrosis, also loses hydration, causing it to become brittle and so more susceptible to tears and ruptures. In a great many cases, this process does not cause any ill effects whatsoever, but in others it can lead to varying degrees of pain, inflammation and loss of flexibility.

Where pain is associated with degenerative disc disease, it typically comes from two sources. First of all, the proteins in the disc space can cause a good deal of inflammation and secondly the outer ring of the disc, as it becomes damaged or worn, becomes less effective in terms of resisting motion in the spine and so causes slight instability. The result can be lower back pain which radiates into the hips or travels down the backs of the legs, stiffness and what can be painful muscle spasms. In addition, if the ligaments and facet joints enlarge to try and compensate for the discs by spreading the load over a wider area, the spinal canal can begin to narrow, compressing the spinal cord and causing nerve pain too.

Particularly when degenerative disc disease starts when a person is still young, it can be a great source of concern as they are left wondering just how much worse it is likely to get with age. The prognosis, however, is actually very good, both because treatment is normally very effective and because the condition often gets better

rather than worse over time. Once the disc has completely degener-
ated, it no longer contains the proteins which cause inflammation and
lead to pain, and so generally it will just collapse into a stable position
and the pain will either lessen or cease altogether.

Conservative treatment options for degenerative disc disorder are
almost always the first to be tried and in most cases these are very
successful. While medications are likely to be prescribed for pain
relief and to help take down any inflammation, physiotherapy may
also be recommended as an additional means of alleviating pain.
Exercise and manipulative treatments, meanwhile, can increase flexibility in the spine, as well as helping to widen the small canals
through which the nerve roots exit the spinal cord.

If surgery should become necessary due to high levels of pain
which remain inadequately addressed by conservative treatments,
then fusion is the most likely option. Basically this works by
stopping any movement in the painful area of the spine, but its effectiveness compared to conservative treatments is as yet unproven.

Because so many people suffer from degenerative disc disease
without experiencing any associated pain, this does make getting a
correct diagnosis very important. In some cases it can be all too easy
for doctors to assume that back pain is the result of this condition
when in fact it could be being caused by something altogether
different. Always be sure, therefore, to choose a physician who specialises in back pain to diagnose and treat the problem.

Facet joint syndrome

Although osteoarthritis is one of the most common culprits in terms
of causing problems with the facet joints in the spine, it is not the only
one. Both injury and other types of degeneration can cause the pain
and stiffness which is typical of facet joint syndrome.

The facet joints, whose technical term is the zygapophysial joints,
are the joints which link each of the vertebrae to the ones above and
below. Not only do they provide strength, stability and flexibility to
the spine, but they also work to limit any excessive movement which
might cause damage to it. Occurring in pairs, they are situated on
either side of the spinal column and their surfaces are covered by a
special type of tissue which is known as articular cartilage. The

joints are lined by a membrane called the synovium and they are enclosed in a fibrous sac known as a joint capsule. The joints are also surrounded by a thick liquid called synovial fluid which acts as lubrication and lets the bones move without friction.

Acute pain which stems from the facet joints can often be the result of a sudden or excessive movement which essentially causes trauma to the joint. This can lead to swelling, inflammation and pain in the joint which might last for several days. More often though, facet joint syndrome is a chronic condition which is caused by longer-term changes in the joint such as might be caused by degenerative disc disease or osteoarthritis. In addition, it might be the result of excessive use of the spine which has caused exceptional levels of deterioration in the discs and in turn affected the facet joints. Athletes such as gymnasts and acrobats are just some of those who are particularly prone to this type of damage.

The pain which is fairly typical of facet joint syndrome tends to occur only on one side of the spine. Bending the spine sideways towards the affected side, bending backwards or straightening the back all tend to aggravate the discomfort and, where a nerve is affected, the symptoms of sciatica may also be experienced with pains travelling through the buttocks, down the legs and stopping just below the knee. Stiffness and limited mobility which tend to feel worse in the mornings are also characteristic of the condition.

Cases of acute facet joint syndrome generally respond well to a treatment programme which includes medication, heat therapy and/ or acupuncture to control pain, drugs to reduce inflammation and physical therapy to increase mobility and flexibility. In addition, conservative treatment courses are also quite likely to include postural correction techniques, as poor posture is believed to play a major role in the development of the condition, as well as recommendations for modifying activities so that they do not involve excessive twisting, stretching or bending.

Chronic facet joint syndrome can sometimes be slightly difficult to diagnose and treat, but where the problem is thought to come directly from the joint, what is known as a facet joint block is often an effective tool for achieving both diagnosis and treatment. A facet joint block involves injecting a local anaesthetic and anti-inflammatory medicine into or close to the nerves which supply the joint. If there is more than a 50% decrease in pain levels, then it can be reliably assumed that the joint is the source of the problem and the procedure can be repeated at a later date as the effects wear off.

Sometimes, however, a longer-term treatment might be required and this is typically achieved through the use of a technique called radiofrequency denervation. This technique involves placing a needle with a small electrode into the facet joint and using an electric current to destroy the nerves. While this method is very effective in terms of pain relief, however, in cases where there is an underlying condition which is causing degeneration of the joint, it will do nothing to either stop or reverse this.

Generally, the outlook for people suffering from facet joint syndrome is good. Conservative treatments are often all that are required for patients to achieve a pain-free existence, and those who have facet joint blocks tend to experience good to excellent pain relief lasting for several months in around 80% of cases.

Failed fusion and adjacent segment degeneration

One of the types of surgery that is relatively common for dealing with neck and back problems which fail to respond to conservative treatments is fusion. This procedure has been performed for many years and, in the vast majority of cases, it is extremely successful. Because fusion requires the bones to knit or 'fuse' together though, something which relies, amongst other things, on the patient not putting too much strain on the spine during the recovery period, there are times when the fusion fails. When this happens, it is known as failed fusion or pseudoarthrosis. It is not a cause of neck or back pain in the same way as the other conditions that I have described, but because the operation effectively fails, it does mean that the pain caused by the original condition continues.

Pseudoarthrosis tends to happen in patients who are considered to be at high risk due to having experienced or because they are currently experiencing a number of other medical problems or because they are smokers. The relevance of smoking in this type of procedure lies in the fact that the nicotine in their bloodstream affects the small blood vessels which are critical to the bone healing process and the formation of bone.

Typically, it takes six to nine months for bones to fuse properly after surgery and of course during this time the patient will be advised to avoid or restrict certain activities such as those which involve lifting, bending or twisting. Even if all due care is taken, however, the bones still may not fuse as they should, in which case a re-operation can be carried out.

Another problem which can arise from spinal fusions is something called adjacent segment degeneration, which basically refers to the degeneration of an intervertebral disc either above or below vertebrae which have previously been fused together. Because there is increased pressure being placed on these discs and they have to absorb more shock, they have a tendency to suffer greater and faster wear and tear than other discs.

Maintaining the natural balance and curvature of the spine when carrying out spinal fusions is vital but tricky, something which is evidenced by the incidence of adjacent segment degeneration. Concern about the condition, however, has since led to the development of artificial disc replacement technology which does away with the need for fusion surgery in cases where there is damage to intervertebral discs. Initial studies seem to suggest that this type of technology may well decrease the risk of adjacent discs incurring damage of their own.

Herniated or 'slipped' disc

A 'herniated disc' is probably more commonly known as a 'slipped disc', but it has to be said that the latter terminology is somewhat misleading. If a doctor diagnoses a 'slipped disc', it is important to understand that nothing in the spine has actually slipped out of place, but there has been damage to one of the intervertebral discs.

Like a bulging disc, a herniated or 'slipped' disc can simply be a result of the aging process and the gradual loss of elasticity in the wall of the disc, making those of middle age or older more susceptible than those in younger age categories. Disc herniation, however, can also be caused by sudden trauma to the spine such as might be experienced in a fall, as the result of a sports injury or by lifting or carrying something awkwardly. Even in these cases, however, it is still those who are over the age of 30 who are most at risk, due to the inherent effects of age, and particularly if they are often involved in strenuous activity.

Rather than the intervertebral disc merely bulging so that it no longer aligns with the vertebra, when a disc herniates, a portion of it actually pushes outside its normal boundary so that it looks like an external bubble. As this bubble protrudes into the spinal canal where there is limited space, it can then begin to press against the nerves of the spine producing severe pain. In the vast majority of cases, disc herniations occur in the more vulnerable lumbar region, with cervical herniations being much less common and thoracic herniations even rarer still.

The extent to which the spinal nerves are being pressurised or pinched will, of course, determine the degree of pain which is experienced, as will the location of the herniation. Pain though, is not the only symptom which may be felt. As I explained earlier, when nerves become compressed or pinched, they can either send out abnormal signals or, sometimes, no signals at all. Patients suffering from herniated discs, therefore, might experience sensations such as electric shock pains, tingling, numbness and muscle weakness. In the case of herniations in the cervical spine, not only might these sensations be felt in the neck itself, but also down the arms. When the lumbar spine is affected, shocks, tingling and so on may also be felt in the legs.

Particularly serious symptoms come in the form of the loss of bladder or bowel control, the sensation of numbness in the area of the genitals or progressive numbness or weakness of the legs. These symptoms can be a sign of cauda equina syndrome, which occurs as a direct result of compression and irritation of the nerves in the lower region of the spinal canal and requires emergency diagnosis and treatment. In some cases, emergency surgery may be required to relieve the pressure on the affected nerves and so avoid the damage becoming permanent.

Although different physicians do take different approaches to the treatment of herniated discs, with the exception of cases involving suspected cauda equina syndrome, most prefer to begin with conservative treatments before proceeding with surgery. Medication to relieve pain and reduce inflammation, bed rest and restrictions to activities which are likely to aggravate the condition, heat or ice therapies, physical therapies such as massage or traction and gentle stretching exercises may all be prescribed in the first instance, but ultimately if these do little or nothing to reduce pain or muscle weakness is increasing, then surgery will very likely become necessary.

There are actually several different types of surgery which can be used to deal with herniated discs, one of the least invasive of which is the micro-laminotomy. This technique involves the surgeon removing a small part of the lamina (part of the spinal ring which covers the spinal cord and nerves) using tiny instruments so that large incisions are not required. Essentially, this technique does not actually repair the damaged disc, but rather provides more room for the herniation and reduces the pressure on the nerve, so alleviating the pain. The surgery normally requires a one or two day stay in hospital for the wound to heal and for post-operative physical therapy to commence, but patients can normally expect any pain in the leg to be resolved immediately and any discomfort in the lower back as a result of the surgery to disappear in anything from a few days to a couple of weeks.

A further type of surgery which is used to treat herniated discs is the discectomy, which basically involves removing the 'bubble' which has escaped into the spinal canal. Generally, this type of surgery takes around an hour to perform under general anaesthetic and involves making an incision in the back which is around three centimetres in length. Again, a one or two night stay in hospital is required and, although leg pain often disappears immediately, it normally takes several weeks for back pain and the pain around the incision to be completely resolved.

Any type of surgery to treat herniated discs, however, is unnecessary in around 90% of cases, with conservative treatment usually being perfectly sufficient to resolve the problem and allow a return to normal activities. In a small number of cases where disc degeneration has led to herniation though, the prognosis can be poorer, with severe and even incapacitating back pain developing and work and life activities being badly affected. Those who have suffered herniation of a disc and are treated with surgery are also statistically more likely to experience the same problem in the same disc. Essentially, in cases where sufferers make little or no effort to address issues such as excess weight, physical conditioning, the nature or way of going about their work and their behavioural activities, the same area of the spine continues to be susceptible to further damage.

Kyphosis

Although it might appear so outwardly, the human spine is not straight but has four natural curves in the cervical, thoracic, lumbar and sacral regions of the neck and back. Disease, developmental disorders, injury or poor posture, however, can mean that what are normally quite gentle curves are more pronounced.

Postural kyphosis

Kyphosis is the term which is used to describe an exaggerated or abnormal curvature of the spine. Postural kyphosis, which affects the middle section of the spine in the thoracic region, is the most common type. The most frequent cause of postural kyphosis is slouching and it is generally during adolescence that the condition starts to become noticeable, with more girls being affected than boys. Rarely, however, does it cause any pain and the vertebrae and the discs all appear perfectly normal. In the majority of cases it can be reversed by correcting imbalances in the muscles through physical therapy so that few, if any, problems are experienced in adulthood.

Postural kyphosis, however, can also occur in older people as a result of degenerative diseases such as arthritis. Compression fractures of the vertebrae caused by osteoporosis or by trauma to the spine are also responsible for the rounded or hunchbacked appearance which is typical of those with kyphosis, and in fact it is estimated that around one third of the most serious cases (known as hyperkyphosis) involve vertebral fractures.

In its most severe form, postural kyphosis gives rise to what is commonly known as a 'dowager's hump' and, when the condition becomes so advanced it can not only cause tremendous discomfort but also restrict normal breathing. Pain and stiffness in the back, as well as muscle fatigue, are some of the most normal symptoms of kyphosis, but in cases where the spinal cord becomes compressed, the numbness, weakness and loss of bladder and bowel control associated with cauda equina syndrome can also be experienced.

Scheuermann's kyphosis

Like postural kyphosis, Scheuermann's kyphosis, or Scheuermann's disease as it is frequently known, is another form of the condition which tends to exhibit itself during adolescence, although in this case sufferers cannot consciously correct their posture. Rather than slouching being the cause of the problem, the disease causes healthy vertebrae which would normally be rectangular to become wedge-shaped so that the upper part of the body curls forwards. Usually it is the thoracic spine which is affected, but it can also occur in the lumbar area. Although the precise cause of the disease is unknown, many believe that the vertebrae develop and grow abnormally and the condition commonly runs in families.

Not only does Scheuermann's kyphosis look much more extreme than postural kyphosis in adolescents, but it also causes severe back pain, particularly when the sufferer takes part in physical activity or stands or sits for prolonged periods of time. With the head and neck being forced into a forwards posture and the individual finding it extremely difficult to stand erect, not only can breathing become laboured, but chest pain can be a problem and even the hamstring muscles in the legs can be caused to tighten. Fatigue is another common symptom of the disease, and this is thought to be due to the fact that the muscles have to work so hard for the sufferer to even be able to sit or stand properly.

Congenital kyphosis

Less common than either postural or Scheuermann's kyphosis is congenital kyphosis, which occurs when the spinal column does not develop properly prior to birth. Usually it is seen in infants, but it can also appear quite suddenly in adolescents, although this is generally in cases where the individual suffers additionally from some kind of neurological disorder such as cerebral palsy. There may be malformation of the vertebrae, or some may even be fused together and, as the child grows, the kyphosis can become progressively worse. Although the risk to the child clearly has to be weighed up in advance, sometimes surgery is required at a very early age to correct the curvature of the spine, with the patient being monitored closely and at regular intervals to assess any changes.

Cervical kyphosis

Kyphosis, as well as affecting the thoracic or middle part of the spine and the lumbar or lower section, can also cause problems in the neck. Looked at from the side, the vertebrae which run from the base of the skull into the upper part of the back would normally curve forwards slightly, but in the case of cervical kyphosis, not only does that curve begin to straighten, but it can even progress to the point where it reverses.

Various things can cause cervical kyphosis, including the degeneration of the vertebral discs, injuries such as those resulting in whiplash, compression fractures or dislocations of the spine, spinal infections and diseases such as osteoporosis. In addition, it can occur as the result of certain congenital diseases. Whatever the cause, however, it is the damage to the vertebrae, facet joints, ligaments and/ or soft tissues of the neck which essentially cause the weight of the head to be inadequately supported, allowing it to be pulled forwards and downwards by the force of gravity.

The degree of pain or the severity of other symptoms associated with cervical kyphosis can vary considerably according to the extent of the condition. Severe pain can be experienced in the neck, shoulders and head as the sufferer attempts to keep the head held upright and movement of the neck can become very limited. In very serious cases, the kyphosis can also put pressure on the roots of the spinal nerves or even directly on the spinal cord itself, causing weakness in the arms or legs and the inability to grip properly, as well as difficulties in walking. Again, in very severe cases, bladder and bowel function can also be affected, in which case immediate medical attention should be sought in order to avoid what could result in paralysis from the neck downwards.

$\sim$

Alongside the physical pain and discomfort associated with the condition, one of the most distressing effects of kyphosis is the change that it brings about to the sufferer's physical appearance. For adolescents in particular, this can severely impact on their self-confidence and their emotional and psychological well-being. In terms of treatment, much depends on the type of kyphosis and the severity of the condition. In the case of congenital kyphosis, for instance, early surgical intervention is often recommended and usually produces the best results, with conservative treatments having little effect. In other types of the condition, if the spinal nerve roots or the spinal column are compromised, then again surgery may be necessary. However, in most cases conservative treatments can be extremely effective in terms of controlling pain, improving mobility and strength and addressing posture and movement so that the effects of the kyphosis are minimised. In some cases, the wearing of a back or neck brace may also help to control the deformity that the condition causes.

Lordosis

In just the same way that a small degree of kyphotic or outward curvature is perfectly normal in the thoracic and sacral regions of the human spine, so a slight inward curvature is natural in the cervical and lumbar regions. Sometimes, however, this curvature is exaggerated in the lower back, a condition which is known in medical terms as lordosis, although more commonly referred to as swayback, saddle back or hollow back.

Like kyphosis, lordosis can occur for a variety of reasons, ranging from developmental disorders and degenerative conditions of the spine to spinal infections, trauma and even excessive weight. Some women also develop a temporary form of the condition during pregnancy, and sitting for extended periods of time at a desk, in a car or on a sofa can also be responsible. In most mild or even moderate cases of lordosis, the individual may feel no negative effects whatsoever, but in more severe cases it can be responsible for a great deal of lower back pain and limited back movement.

Because the vertebrae which make up the various sections of the spine are all connected, conditions which affect one area can sometimes have a knock-on effect on other areas and so it is not uncommon to see kyphosis of the thoracic spine and lordosis of the lumbar spine in the same patient. This in itself, however, does not necessarily mean that the individual will experience greater levels of pain and, as stated previously, it is generally only more exaggerated curvatures which cause troublesome symptoms.

Treatment of lordosis is not normally necessary unless it is causing pain or other problematic symptoms, such as might be the case if nerves become constricted or there is limited movement. Where this is the case, over-the-counter pain medication may be recommended or stronger painkillers prescribed, as well as anti-inflammatory drugs where necessary. Physical therapy, meanwhile, can do much to strengthen back muscles and improve mobility and a back brace may help to control posture and stop the progression of the curve, although long-term use can have detrimental effects on the back muscles. Where excessive weight has caused or contributed to the problem, then an appropriate weight loss diet and exercise regime may also be recommended.

In severe cases where conservative treatments are ineffective, surgery may be required to correct the curvature. The commonest surgical treatment used for the condition is spinal fusion, but as this can lead to degeneration in other areas of the spine (see earlier section on adjacent segment degeneration), this solution would generally only be used as a last resort.

Lumbago

Lumbago is not so much a direct cause of back pain as an umbrella term which is used to refer to general pain in the lower part of the back. The pain might originate from any number of sources but often the exact cause is unknown. It might, for instance, be the result of a strain caused by heavy lifting, although problems with the intervertebral discs, osteoporosis, arthritis, tumours and a variety of other causes all can and should be identified.

Lumbago is actually very common, and most people will experience at least one episode of lower back pain during the course of their lives. Around 90% of those individuals will make a complete recovery within about six weeks, but for those whose pain continues it is important to seek a proper diagnosis and treatment from a specialist in back disorders.

Sincce the causes of lumbago are so wide-ranging, obviously the extent of the pain and the type of pain can be highly variable. With so many different anatomical structures in the back, including muscles, ligaments, tendons, bones, facet joints, discs and nerves, there is certainly plenty that can go wrong, but it is important to remember that the severity of the pain does not necessarily equate to the seriousness of the problem. A simple strain from twisting suddenly or lifting something heavy, for example, can lead to pain which is far more excruciating than that caused by a herniated disc.

Not only do levels of pain vary across different causes of back pain, but also across individuals. Two people might suffer the same condition but experience entirely different levels of symptoms. While one might be perfectly able to continue with normal daily activities, the other could be completely incapacitated. It is for this reason that professional physicians who are experienced in back pain will treat each and every case in its own right and will tailor the treatment to the individual.

Expert diagnosis though, is extremely important, and those who suffer from back pain should never allow themselves to be palmed off with a diagnosis of lumbago. Because the treatments which are appropriate for different underlying causes vary, it is essential to identify the real source of the problem.

In most cases of lower back pain, conservative, non-surgical treatments are extremely effective in terms of relieving pain and other symptoms, even when those symptoms are chronic. Only in rarer cases is it necessary for surgical procedures to be carried out and generally this would only be done if conservative treatments proved to be unsuccessful.

Muscle tension

While staying off the roads and the rugby field might afford some form of protection from injuries to the neck and back, even those whose lifestyles are much more sedentary can still be at risk of suffering neck and back pain. Everyday activities such as watching television or reading can place strain or tension on the neck muscles if posture is poor. Working on a computer for hours on end when the monitor is placed significantly above or below eye level can also cause problems, as can bending over a desk for hours, painting a ceiling or sleeping in an awkward position. Essentially, anything which involves either repetitive movements, overuse of muscles or prolonged immobilisation can lead to muscle tension and associated pain and inflammation of the soft tissues.

Stress too plays an enormous role in creating neck and back pain as these areas of the body are particularly sensitive to its effects. The act of tensing muscles when we feel stressed not only restricts the flow of blood to the body's tissues, and with it the flow of oxygen and nutrients, but it also prevents the body from effectively flushing out acidic waste from the muscles. The build-up of this waste not only leads to pain, but also fatigue.

Stress also leaves us more vulnerable to injury because muscles which are tensed respond differently to even normal things such as sitting for too long, twisting or lifting something slightly heavy. Where a person is already suffering from neck or back pain, stress and the increasing tensing of muscles can add to the severity of the symptoms and so begins a vicious cycle.

Of course, as with any case of neck or back pain, ruling out other potential causes is essential if the correct treatment is to be applied, and so it is important to consult an expert who specialises in these types of conditions. Once muscle tension has been identified as either the cause of the pain or the aggravating factor, however, the next step is to work on relieving the tension and correct the situation or behaviour which has led to the problem. This might be approached, for example, by improving posture and the ways in which the body is used, or by rearranging work spaces and investing in ergo-nomically designed furniture.

Massage, and especially deep tissue massage, can be especially useful in helping to break down tight muscles, while manipulative treatments can be very effective in terms of improving mobility. Heat therapy, meanwhile, can offer considerable benefits by helping to reduce pain and encouraging relaxation, and working on strength-ening muscles can do much to support improved posture. When you work alongside your specialist physician, he or she will provide a full assessment of your condition which will take into account your lifestyle and behaviours and will help him or her to make a correct diagnosis and prescribe an effective treatment programme.

Myelopathy

Myelopathy is a term which is used to describe the gradual loss of nerve function due to dysfunction of the spinal cord. Sometimes this happens directly as the result of a spinal injury, such as that which might occur in a motoring or sports-related accident, whereas in other cases it is degenerative disease which is responsible for the complete or partial loss of sensation and movement.

Myelopathy can occur in the cervical, thoracic or lumbar regions of the spine. In the cervical region it will typically affect the upper limbs, wrists and hands and, the higher up the cervical spine the damage occurs, the greater the effect. Serious injuries to the upper cervical spine can also affect breathing and so may require immediate medical intervention.

In the thoracic and lumbar regions, meanwhile, the loss of movement or feeling is experienced in the legs, hips, bladder, bowels and sexual functions, and in some cases these too need to be treated as a medical emergency. Where the injury is to the upper thoracic region, the upper abdomen, lower chest and various internal processes can also be affected. In the most serious cases of myelopathy caused by injury, almost all of the systems of the body can be impaired and patients can be left unable to walk, use their arms or even control their breathing without assistance from a ventilator.

One of the commonest causes of myelopathy which is not related to injury is a condition called spinal stenosis, which most often affects the lower back or neck. This condition, which will be discussed in more detail a little later on, essentially involves a general compression and narrowing of the spinal column which leads to the nerves being pinched. Where it occurs in the neck (cervical stenosis), it is often the pain in the arms which leads patients to seek a diagnosis from a qualified practitioner. Even conditions such as herniated discs though, can cause dysfunction of the spinal cord. As might be expected, in most cases involving degenerative diseases of the neck and back, myelopathy occurs much more gradually than with spinal injuries, but it still produces, to a greater or lesser extent, weakness or altered sensation in the limbs, random or spasmodic movements and even incontinence.

Many of the people who suffer from myelopathy as a result of degenerative disorders tend to be older. Because their bodies are naturally slowing down anyway, this can make the detection of the characteristic signs of the condition, including weakness, lack of responsiveness and changes in co-ordination, difficult. If there has been a long history of neck pain or recent changes in terms of co-ordination abilities and so on, however, it is always wise to have these checked out.

Because myelopathy is related to pressure on the nerves in the spine, surgery is often offered much sooner than in the case of some other neck and back complaints. One of the difficulties with frail or elderly patients, however, is that the operation itself represents a risk and so the benefits of surgery need to be weighed against this. Where the risk is considered to be too great or surgery is not the preferred option, there are though, conservative treatments which can offer significant relief for the symptoms, including physical therapy, traction, massage, heat therapy and electrical stimulation, as well as a variety of pain relief medications, muscle relaxants and anti-inflammatory drugs.

Osteoporosis

Osteoporosis is a condition which causes the bones to thin and lose their density over time, essentially making them weaker, more fragile and much more susceptible to injury. It is what might be called a 'silent' disease in the respect that typically there are no warning signs of the condition and it is only when the first fracture is experienced that people become aware of it.

Although the cause of the disease is still as yet unknown, it is believed that most of the 50% of women and the 20% of men over 50 in the UK who experience a fracture will do so as a result of osteoporosis, which is thought to affect some 3 million people in the UK.

The loss of bone density is actually a natural process of ageing which starts at around the age of 35. As we grow older, our bones grow increasingly less able to repair and regenerate themselves and so the mesh of tiny struts of bone which form a honeycomb inside the hard outer shell begins to get less dense. In some people, and particularly post-menopausal women, this can lead to osteoporosis and the increased risk of fracture. The disease can, however, also affect men, younger women and even children, especially if they also suffer from chronic rheumatoid arthritis, chronic kidney disease or eating disorders or if they have been taking corticosteroid medications every day for a period of more than three months. Those who have been confined to bed due to accident or illness for considerable lengths of time are also at higher risk of developing the condition.

The three parts of the body which are most affected by fractures due to osteoporosis are the wrists, the hips and the spine, and a recent report suggested that in India, a massive 83% of all spinal fractures happen as a result of the disease. The lumbar and thoracic regions of the spine are most commonly affected by vertebral fractures which essentially cause the bones to become crushed or compressed. As described previously, these compression fractures are typically wedge-shaped and do not usually interfere with the spinal cord but, if they are numerous and are not corrected with surgery, they can cause a permanent loss of height as well as curvature of the spine. If the latter is serious enough, the reduced amount of space available for the internal organs can cause shortness of breath, digestion problems, the protrusion of the stomach and stress incontinence.

Because the bones of people with osteoporosis can in some cases be so brittle, it does not necessarily take very much for fractures to occur. Lifting a heavy shopping bag or reaching up to a high shelf, for example, can be enough to cause one or more vertebrae to fracture, and even an episode of coughing or sneezing can be sufficient to cause damage. When this happens, lower back or neck pain are normally the symptoms which are experienced, depending on which of the vertebrae have been affected.

The disease though, does not slow down or stop the healing process of broken bones and most will heal quite successfully on their own within eight to twelve weeks. In the meantime, any associated pain or inflammation can be treated with medication. In addition to pain-killing and anti-inflammatory drugs, however, there is also a range of different drug treatments which are aimed at reducing the risk of future fractures by strengthening the bones.

Exercise and diet are two other big considerations when it comes to treating osteoporosis. Weight-bearing and resistance exercises which are carried out regularly can help to reduce the likelihood of bone fractures and a diet which is high in calcium, vitamin D (which helps the body to absorb calcium) and protein will help to keep the body supplied with the essential ingredients that it needs to form and maintain a healthy bone structure.

The outlook for patients with osteoporosis is extremely variable and some can even become severely disabled or die after having sustained fractures as a result of the disease. The vast majority of these more serious cases, however, involve people who have suffered fractures of the hip rather than within the spine. Only around half of those with hip fractures regain full mobility and independence, and the mortality rate for older patients is reported to be around 20% at three months, although many of these deaths are caused by complications such as deep vein thrombosis or pneumonia.

In the case of vertebral fractures, while patients who have suffered one compression fracture are up to five times more likely to suffer a further one, in some cases they may not even be aware of the damage that has been sustained. Generally though, some degree of ongoing pain is likely to be experienced and this can, in some cases, be severe. Pain management methods and conservative treatments, however, can do much to reduce pain and restore quality of life. Where there are multiple fractures, this can result in a pronounced curvature of the spine called kyphosis (commonly known as a 'dowager's hump' or 'hunch back') and pressure on internal organs which can make it difficult to breathe. These cases, however, are rare.

Other medical conditions

The various causes of neck and back pain which have been described so far, as well as the ones that you will read about in the rest of this chapter, all originate directly from the various structures of the neck and back, such as the muscles, joints, nerves and bones. There are, however, a number of other medical conditions which can cause pain in these areas, albeit from completely different sources, amongst them fibromyalgia, lower urinary tract infections, the kidney infection known as pyelonephritis, kidney stones and endometriosis.

Fibromyalgia

Fibromyalgia is an extremely common and yet baffling condition which is believed to bring misery to literally hundreds of millions of people across the world, around 80 to 90% of whom are women. It typically brings with it a whole range of symptoms, including severe and persistent fatigue, sleep disturbances, headaches and cognitive and memory impairment (often referred to as fibro fog or brain fog), but its main characteristics are musculoskeletal pain, tenderness of the soft tissues, stiffness of the muscles, tendons and ligaments, muscle spasms, numbness and tingling, all of which can appear just about anywhere in the body.

As you can see, many of these latter symptoms are ones which are also present in cases where injuries to the back or neck have been sustained, or where some type of degenerative disease of the spine is present. As there is no single test which can categorically identify fibromyalgia, however, this can make diagnosis extremely difficult and doctors frequently rely quite heavily on a process of elimination when trying to decide whether fibromyalgia is in fact the cause of the symptoms. As there are dozens of other conditions which can cause similar symptoms though, and the aches and pains which are typically experienced in fibromyalgia can move around from one part of the body to another from day to day, this can often be a long, drawn-out process during which patients typically become increasingly fearful and frustrated.

The musculoskeletal pain which tends to be one of the most significant symptoms of fibromyalgia can affect any of 18 separate muscle groups in the body. Along with the shoulders, pelvic region and hands, however, it is the neck and back which are most often affected. Although the pain actually comes from the muscles, tendons and ligaments, patients describe it as originating in the joints and so it can easily be confused with the pain associated with arthritis. Sharp, stabbing pains and deep muscular aches, which are often more noticeable when the muscles are being used, can also appear to signify some kind of physiological damage to the structures of the back or neck, but in fact there is no detectable damage to the body in fibromyalgia at all, which is why there are still some doctors today who consider the condition to be 'all in the mind'.

As well as the more widespread musculoskeletal pain experienced by fibromyalgia sufferers, there is also a tenderness of the soft tissues of the body. When even the slightest pressure is applied to these 'tender points', sometimes even extreme levels of pain can be felt. In fact, it is these tender points which are used as one of the factors for determining the presence of fibromyalgia when doctors are carrying out a diagnosis. If widespread pain has been experienced in all four quadrants of the body (on both sides of the body and above and below the waist) for at least three months and if at least 11 out of the 18 recognised tender points around the body respond with a painful reaction, then the patient would qualify for a diagnosis of the condition. Interestingly though, most of these tender points are located in the area of the neck and shoulders, which again can make diagnosis somewhat tricky.

Stiffness of the muscles, tendons and ligaments is another symptom of fibromyalgia which can cause it to be confused with problems originating directly from the neck or back. When patients begin to find it difficult to sit or stand comfortably for any length of time without it causing stiffness of the back, it is quite natural to assume that this is the result of a strain or a disc problem, when in fact fibromyalgia may well be the cause. In addition, the numbness and tingling, particularly in the arms, legs, hands and feet, which is typical of fibromyalgia, could very easily be interpreted as the more worrying symptom of damage to the nerves in the spine. Muscle spasms in the back, legs and buttocks, meanwhile, might at first appear to be entirely characteristic of sciatica, but in fact have nothing to do with the sciatic nerve at all.

Whilst various hypotheses have been put forward in relation to the cause of fibromyalgia, it still remains a mystery to the medical profession. Some think it is down to a dysfunction of the central nervous system or chemical or hormonal imbalances in the body, while others believe that there is a genetic connection or that environmental factors are to blame. Others still are convinced that trauma or injury is responsible for the condition, and it is perhaps in the case of whiplash injuries to the neck where there is the greatest potential for confusion, as studies have shown that a high proportion of cases of fibromyalgia are in fact triggered in this way.

The prognosis for sufferers of fibromyalgia in terms of a cure are currently not good because without being able to identify a categorical cause of the condition, finding a cure is, of course, impossible. As with most other conditions which cause or contribute to neck or back pain, however, there is a great deal that can be done in terms of conservative treatments to provide significant relief and help to restore a decent quality of life.

The most effective approach to treating fibromyalgia has proven to be a holistic and multidisciplinary one which might not only involve the prescription of medications such as analgesics, muscle relaxants or antidepressants, but also incorporates a programme of exercise, a range of physiotherapy techniques such as massage and perhaps psychotherapy or cognitive behavioural therapy to help deal with underlying issues which may be contributing to the stress, anxiety and depression which are commonly factors associated with the condition. A whole range of alternative remedies and treatments such as herbal remedies and supplements of certain vitamins and essential elements have also proven to be highly effective in many cases.

Something else which is key to treating and managing the often devastating effects of fibromyalgia are certain changes to lifestyle. Because particular elements of an individual's diet can quite often trigger symptoms or cause them to worsen, identifying problem foods and eliminating these from the diet can have remarkable effects. Attending to posture and sleep routines, as well as avoiding or managing stress are also important considerations, and even simple things like taking sufficient rest, pacing oneself and writing things down can do much to help with the varying symptoms of fibromyalgia.

Lower urinary tract infections

Urinary tract infections, or UTIs as they are more commonly known, are believed to be the second most common type of infection to affect the human body and can cause a range of unpleasant symptoms which might include lower back or abdominal pain.

Starting from the top, the urinary system is comprised of the kidneys, ureters, bladder and urethra. Amongst other things, the kidneys are responsible for removing waste products and excess liquid from the body by filtering them through the blood. The urine which they produce is then carried down from the kidneys to the bladder via two narrow tubes called ureters, where it is stored until such time as the bladder is emptied and then released through the urethra. Ordinarily, the bacteria which live in the bowel, on the skin near the rectum and in the vagina do not interfere with the normal functioning of the urinary system, but if these bacteria enter the urethra and begin to travel upwards, they can cause infection in the bladder, as well as in other parts of the urinary tract. Women are notoriously more susceptible to these types of infections, something which many believe to be down to the fact that they have a shorter urinary tract than men.

Often some of the first things that those experiencing urinary tract infections will be aware of are the urge to urinate more frequently, the feeling of needing to urinate again immediately after the bladder has been emptied and a painful, burning sensation whilst passing urine. The urine itself typically has a strong odour, looks cloudy or contains signs of blood. In addition, however, these symptoms are often accompanied by lower back or abdominal pain in the area of the bladder and, occasionally the patient will show signs of fever. Because the symptoms of UTIs often appear quite suddenly, however, back pain may well be an early indicator of this type of problem.

Lower urinary tract infections are normally treated with a simple course of antibiotics, but it is important to get symptoms checked out at the earliest opportunity before the infection has the chance to spread to the kidneys and the condition becomes much more serious.

Pyelonephritis
Particularly where urinary tract or bladder infections remain untreated, the infection can travel upwards to affect usually one, although occasionally both kidneys, resulting in what can be a serious kidney infection called pyelonephritis. Sometimes, however, pyelonephritis can develop without there having been a bladder infection, such as in cases where there is an abnormality of the kidney or where there are kidney stones present.

Although it is usually the case that someone with pyelonephritis will experience the sensation of needing to pass urine often or pain when urinating, this does not always happen. Pain, however, either in the side of the abdomen or in the area of the back above the kidney, along with a high temperature, nausea, vomiting and/or diarrhoea and possibly blood in the urine, are normally good indicators of a kidney infection. If this is suspected, it is important to visit a doctor as soon as possible for testing and treatment as complications such as kidney damage and septicaemia (a serious and potentially even life-threatening infection of the blood otherwise known as 'blood poisoning') can occur.

The test that doctors use to diagnose pyelonephritis is a simple dipstick urine test, but often physicians will send off a urine sample to a laboratory to find out precisely what type of bacterium is causing the problem so that the correct type of antibiotics can be prescribed. Treatment in the form of antibiotics, however, will normally begin straight away whilst these test results are being awaited. In addition, painkillers may be prescribed, both to bring down any fever and to deal with any associated pain.

Kidney stones

Although they may not sound particularly horrific, kidney stones can be the cause of excruciating back pain. In cases where these hard masses of crystal remain tiny, and sometimes as small as a grain of sand, they can pass from the kidney and through the urinary tract without a person even knowing about it. When they grow larger, however, and move into the urinary tract, blocking the flow of urine, they can cause pain which some describe as being comparable to natural childbirth. As the muscles in the wall of the ureter try to squeeze the stone through the narrow tube and out into the bladder, there can be sharp, stabbing pains on the side of the affected kidney which may be accompanied by blood in the urine as the body attempts to rid itself of the stone.

Although it is not known precisely what causes kidney stones to form, the most common types are largely made up of calcium, which is of course part of a person's normal diet. As many people remain unaffected by kidney stones throughout their lives, and as they do seem to run in families, it is believed that it is an individual's suscept-ibility which is most significant in their formation, rather than anything to do with what we eat. It may be that the chemicals which are normally contained within urine to prevent the formation of these crystals simply do not work as well for some people as for others. In some rarer cases, it can be an infection in the urinary tract which causes a kidney stone to develop.

For some people, the first sign of a kidney stone might be a very sharp, cramping pain as the stone moves in the urinary tract, but this is not always the case. A dull, continuous or intermittent pain, rather like toothache but experienced in the lower back or pelvis, might persist for hours or even days before becoming more localised and intense. Either way, it might be easy to think that the problem originates from the structures of the back, rather than from the internal organs, espe-cially as other symptoms such as blood in the urine or nausea or vomiting may not be present. In cases where the pain is accompanied by fever and chills, this may indicate the presence of an infection, in which case it is necessary to contact a doctor immediately.

Although some kidney stones grow too large to pass through the urinary system on their own, in most cases this is not the case and drinking plenty of water is usually all that is required to pass them naturally in the urine. Pain medication may also be prescribed to take away the discomfort which is felt in the meantime. Only in cases where stones are much too large to be passed naturally would other types of treatment be considered, the most common of which is extracorporeal shock wave lithotripsy (ESWL) which basically uses shock waves created outside of the body to break down the stones into particles which are small enough to be passed through the urinary tract in the normal way. Particularly large kidney stones, or those which are inaccessible in terms of using ESWL, might have to be surgically removed.

Drinking more water generally, as well as certain dietary changes may be recommended to those people who have already experienced kidney stones and appear to be susceptible to them, in order to try to prevent a recurrence. Certain medications can also be prescribed which help to prevent either calcium-based or uric acid stones from developing in the first place.

Endometriosis

Lower back pain, despite being a common symptom of endometriosis, is one which is nevertheless poorly recognised. Although pelvic pain before and/or after menstruation, severe menstrual cramps, painful intercourse and orgasm, heavy or irregular menstrual bleeding, bladder pain, painful bowel movements and intense fatigue are typically cited as symptoms of the condition, pain in the lower back is less often mentioned but just as often felt.

Endometriosis is a very painful condition in which cells like those which form the lining of the womb (the endometrium) grow elsewhere in the body. Typically they are found on the ovaries, the Fallopian tubes, the outer surface of the uterus or intestines and on the surface lining of the pelvic cavity. Less commonly, they may also be found in the bladder, cervix or vagina. It is a major cause of infertility and one of the main reasons why hysterectomies are carried out.

Endometriosis is so painful because the cells which grow outside the womb behave in precisely the same way as those inside. At the appropriate point in the monthly cycle, the body's hormones stimulate the endometriosis, causing it to grow, break down and bleed. Because the blood has nowhere to go, however, pain, inflammation and adhesions (scar tissue) are the results. Where the back is affected, the pain may not be restricted solely to the lumbar region. Any interference with the sciatic nerve may also cause the pain to extend through the buttocks and down the back of either or both legs.

Although a variety of theories have been put forward to explain the cause of the condition, such as immune dysfunction, genetic predisposition and various environmental causes, none of these has been shown to explain categorically why it occurs and consequently there is, as yet, no known cure. Treatments, therefore, are aimed at relieving pain, shrinking or slowing the growth of the endometriosis and preventing, or at least delaying the recurrence of the disease. Considerable efforts are also made to either restore or preserve fertility.

Like so many other diseases and illnesses, endometriosis affects everyone differently, not least because pain is an extremely personal thing that we each experience differently. In the case of endometriosis, therefore, the extent of the condition does not necessarily correlate with the amount of pain which is felt and so each case needs to be treated separately and on its own merits.

Short-term and immediate relief from the back pain associated with endometriosis can generally be achieved by taking painkillers and anti-inflammatory drugs. Heat therapy can also be very effective at easing back pain in some cases, and the use of a transcutaneous electrical nerve stimulator (TENS) machine may also provide significant relief, as may alternative treatments such as acupuncture. Because the pain is not only severe, but frequent, however, many women require a longer term pain management solution. In some cases, birth control pills may be prescribed. By regulating the hormones within the body, these basically interfere with the messages to the endometrial tissue, telling it to prepare for pregnancy, so making it less likely to break down and bleed. Where more radical treatment is necessary to provide long-term relief, this might range from the less invasive keyhole surgery to remove unwanted cells, to the complete removal of the uterus, Fallopian tubes and ovaries as in a hysterectomy. In some cases, the onset of the menopause will bring about its own natural remedy for the condition.

Pregnancy

As it is not, of course, an illness, pregnancy might seem like an odd thing to include in a list of causes of back pain. As many mothers will know, however, lower back pain during pregnancy can not only be a real problem in the time leading up to the birth, but also during the birth and for what might be a considerable length of time afterwards.

Although it is relatively common, back pain during pregnancy should not just be accepted as a normal part of the process – after all, it is not something which affects every pregnant woman without exception – and so it is always worth seeking expert advice, not least to rule out the possibility of an underlying problem which the sufferer may not previously have been aware of. If nothing else, managing the pain throughout the pregnancy will ensure that the mother, and consequently the baby, is much happier and more relaxed.

Basically, there are two main types of back pain which are commonly experienced during pregnancy, the first of which affects the lower back or lumbar region and the second of which the posterior pelvic region. In the case of the first, pain which is felt at around waist level may or may not be accompanied by that which radiates into the leg or foot. It is generally aggravated by standing or sitting for too long, as well as by repetitive lifting movements and does not feel dissimilar to lower back pain which is experienced by those who are not pregnant. This type of back pain during pregnancy is less common than posterior pelvic pain.

Pain which is felt in the back of the pelvis tends to be a deep pain which is experienced on one or both sides and below the waistline, typically across the tailbone. It may extend into the buttocks and down the backs of the thighs and can also be associated with pubic pain. Lifting, twisting and bending forwards, sitting and rising from a seated position, climbing stairs, running and walking can all trigger or aggravate posterior pelvic pain, as can anything which involves prolonged periods of inactivity, such as sitting at a computer for hours on end.

Of course, not all back pain during pregnancy is a result of the current pregnancy itself. In some cases, an injury or even a previous difficult birth can lead to painful flare-ups when a woman becomes pregnant later on. In many cases, however, it is the changes which occur naturally in the body at this time which are responsible for the problem. While the perfectly normal levels of weight gain can add stress to the back, the fact that most of the weight is carried to the front of the body, something which effectively changes the woman's centre of gravity, can lead to muscular imbalances and muscle fatigue. Surges of pregnancy hormones, meanwhile, can cause the joints to become lax which, when combined with the additional weight and the centre of gravity changes, can mean that the joints become less well supported.

Investigating the source of back pain during pregnancy is, though, important. When experienced in the lower back for several weeks or months, it can be a predictor of post partum back pain, or pain which is experienced after the birth, and so seeking treatment is advised in order to avoid this. Pain which is only experienced post partum should also be thoroughly investigated, otherwise there is the risk that it could become chronic or recur throughout the individual's life.

There is a range of conservative treatments which can be recommended to women suffering from back pain during pregnancy and these would typically concentrate on appropriate exercise, posture and the proper use of body mechanics. Gentle massage of the affected area can also be particularly helpful, but of course great care needs to be taken by pregnant women when it comes to certain medications and herbal remedies. For the sake of your own health and that of your baby, it is always advisable to seek the advice of a medical specialist who is trained and experienced in back problems.

Radiculopathy

Radiculopathy is another one of those terms which is used by doctors to describe symptoms in the neck and back which might originate from a number of different causes. In this case, the pain, tingling, numbness or weakness results from a problem related to the roots of the nerves which connect the spine to the rest of the nervous system, such as might be caused by irritation or compression.

Diseases, infections and injuries can all be responsible for radiculopathy, and in particular those injuries which compress the vertebrae. Herniated discs which put pressure on the nerve roots are another common cause of the condition.

Radiculopathy can affect the cervical, thoracic or lumbar regions of the spine. Usually it creates pain and numbness which radiate out from the spine and can be felt in the arms or legs, although it can also cause hypersensitivity to touch. Weakness of the muscles which are supplied by the nerve is also quite common and, depending on the area which is affected, neck and/or shoulder pain, headaches, muscle stiffness and restricted range of motion may also be experienced. Where the affected nerve is in the lower back, the symptoms are most often those of sciatica, with pain running from the back, through the buttocks and down the backs of the thighs to around knee level. The type of pain and its intensity can however vary, and some might experience a more widespread, dull ache whilst others might feel it as a sharp, burning and more localised pain.

Before the treatment of radiculopathy can begin, it is vital that the underlying cause of the problem be accurately diagnosed by a specialist in neck and back disorders. Although in many cases conservative treatments might be entirely appropriate, this will of course depend on the nature and extent of an injury or disease and so the cause of pain, tingling, numbness or weakness in the neck or back areas should always be thoroughly investigated.

Retrolisthesis

Retrolisthesis is a condition in which one of the vertebrae in the spine slips backwards in relation to the bone above and/or below it. It can actually be thought of as the precise opposite of the condition known as spondylolisthesis in which the vertebra slips forwards. Retrolisthesis, however, is much less common.

In most cases involving adults, retrolisthesis happens because a vertebral disc either deteriorates or ruptures and causes the bone to lose its support, and degenerative diseases such as arthritis are often at the root of the problem. Severe injuries, and particularly those which lead to stress fractures, can also be responsible, as can certain nutritional deficiencies and bad posture. However, in cases where children are affected, it is most often as the result of a congenital spine defect.

Although retrolisthesis can happen at any point along the vertebral column, most cases involve either the cervical or lumbar regions. The severity of any symptoms experienced will depend entirely on where the misalignment of the vertebrae occurs, as well as on the extent of the misalignment. In cases where one vertebra has slipped backwards in relation to the bone immediately above or below it, this is known as partial retrolisthesis, whereas a stair-stepped retrolisthesis occurs when one vertebra moves behind the bone above it but in front of the bone below. Complete retrolisthesis, meanwhile, is where the slipped vertebra is positioned backwards in relation to the bones immediately above and below it.

In cases where the slippage of the vertebra occurs in the lower back, stiffness, constant pain when standing, sitting or walking and limited mobility may all be the result, whereas in the neck it is more likely to be a dull pain and a feeling of tenderness which is experienced. Sensations of pain, however, can depend on how close the misaligned bone comes into contact with either the roots of the spinal nerves or the soft tissue. If it does not come too close to either, then the level of pain tends to be much lower, but in cases where there is pressure on the nerves this can lead to numbness or tingling in the arms, shoulders, neck, legs, hips, buttock or thigh, and even in the torso. In addition, some people who suffer from retrolisthesis have a tendency to compensate for feelings of instability in the back or neck by standing or holding themselves in certain ways, which in itself can cause further problems and restrict their ability to move freely.

If the symptoms of retrolisthesis remain untreated, they tend to worsen over time, and this is especially the case when a degenerative disorder is the cause of the problem. Seeking a sound diagnosis and appropriate treatment is, therefore, very important, and in most cases non-surgical, conservative treatment will be the preferred way forward. Traditional and/or alternative methods of pain relief may be offered to help deal with any discomfort, but in addition, physical therapy can help to return the slipped vertebra to its correct position. Where excessive weight or nutritional deficiencies have caused or contributed to the problem, then these too will be addressed via appropriate diets or supplementation. Only in extreme cases would surgery normally be considered as an option, and the aim of this would be to restore the spine to its proper alignment, usually by carrying out a spinal fusion.

Rheumatoid arthritis

Despite both having the word 'arthritis' in the name, degenerative arthritis, or osteoarthritis as it is also known, and rheumatoid arthritis are in many ways quite different. Most significantly, the former occurs as the result of general wear and tear which causes the breakdown of the joint cartilage, whereas the latter, which is generally a much more severe and chronic condition, is an inflammatory disease in which the immune system begins to attack the body's healthy tissues. While the specific cause of rheumatoid arthritis is not known, both gender and genetics are believed to be important factors in determining an individual's predisposition to the disease, with women being around three times more likely to develop it than men.

Because osteoarthritis occurs due to gradual deterioration within the joints, it is typically those in the older age categories or those whose joints are subjected to repeated stress who suffer its effects.

With rheumatoid arthritis, however, the onset of the disease can start at any age, although there may be periods of remission at certain times. Where osteoarthritis typically begins in a single joint, rheumatoid arthritis usually affects multiple joints at the same time.

Rather than joint cartilage being primarily affected, in rheumatoid arthritis it is the lining of the joint, known as the synovium, which suffers most damage. This membrane becomes severely inflamed and, in severe cases, the condition can destroy joint tissues entirely, including cartilage, ligaments, tendons and bone. In very serious, but thankfully rare cases, it can even cause damage to the body's organs, such as the heart, lungs and skin.

As well as affecting the hands, wrists, elbows, shoulders, knees and feet, rheumatoid arthritis can also cause severe damage to the spine in the neck and back, although particularly in the cervical spine. In fact, one study suggests that as many as 83% of sufferers of the condition experience its effects in the neck within just two years of the onset of the disease. As the joints in the spine are destroyed by rheumatoid arthritis, the connection between each of the vertebrae becomes unstable, allowing the upper vertebra to slide forward on top of the lower one in a process which is known as spondylolisthesis. This slippage can not only cause pressure on nerve roots, but also directly on the spinal cord itself.

Of the seven vertebrae which make up the cervical spine, it is in the top two, C1 and C2, where joint stability is most serious. The C1 or atlas vertebra is the one which basically supports the weight of the head, and the C2 or axis vertebra is the one which helps the atlas to rotate, so giving the neck its incredible range of mobility. Although rheumatoid arthritis can affect the joints in the thoracic and lumbar regions of the spine, this is less common.

Rheumatoid arthritis in the spine affects everyone differently and can present with a wide range of symptoms, which can make it very difficult for doctors to diagnose. Pain, however, is generally the first sign and where the cervical spine is affected, this will typically be felt at the base of the skull. Usually the pain is directly associated with the inflammation of the joint and it may be accompanied by stiffness and decreased ability to bend the neck and turn the head.

As the disease progresses, pain may also be felt elsewhere in the neck and down into the back, but more worrying than the pain are the symptoms which begin to appear with pressure on the spinal cord which could include:

- blackouts caused by pressure on the vertebral arteries as the head and neck are moved in particular ways;
- irregular gait, weakness and problems with balance caused by pressure on the spinal cord;
- tingling, weakness or loss of co-ordination in the arms or legs;
- changes in bladder or bowel control, including incontinence or the inability to urinate.

In some cases, the effects of rheumatoid arthritis on the spine may be minimal, but in others they can be severely disabling and even life-threatening. The pain, swelling and stiffness can eventually lead to loss of function and, after five years, it is estimated that around one third of patients are unable to work. Ten years after the onset of the disease, meanwhile, approximately half of sufferers will have suffered substantial physical disability.

Although spontaneous remission in rheumatoid arthritis is believed to be rare, there is evidence to suggest that treatment can drive the condition into remission as well as controlling the inflammation and minimising the damage to the joints. Any treatment which is administered, however, must be tailored to the individual case, taking into account the severity of symptoms, the response to particular types of therapy and any side effects which might be experienced, such as those to certain medications.

In terms of drug therapy, there are several different types of medication which might be prescribed and these include:

- non-steroidal anti-inflammatory drugs (NSAIDs) to relieve pain and reduce inflammation;
- disease-modifying anti-rheumatic drugs (DMARDs) to reduce inflammation, reduce or prevent damage to the joints and preserve joint structure and function;
- biologic response modifiers to prevent or reduce inflammation;
- steroids to provide fast relief from inflammation, swelling, tenderness, pain and stiffness;

■ painkillers.

In all cases of rheumatoid arthritis, however, treatment needs to extend much further than just medication. Exercise, physical therapies, rest and nutrition and dietary therapies are all key to successfully managing the condition. Because the disease has such enormous potential to affect not only physical, but also mental and psychological well-being, however, education, counselling and cognitive behavioural therapy are just as important in helping sufferers to understand, come to terms with and manage the challenges of their condition.

Where joints have become severely deformed by rheumatoid arthritis or where the compression on spinal nerves needs to be relieved, surgery may be required.

Ruptured disc

A ruptured disc is similar to a herniated disc, but in this case, rather than there just being a protrusion through the wall of the intervertebral disc, the fibrous outer shell actually tears, bursts or breaks and the nucleus pulposus or gelatine-like inner substance leaks into the surrounding tissue. In cases where the rupture occurs under pressure, what typically happens is that part of the ruptured disc prolapses out and compresses the sciatic nerve which runs down the leg, causing severe pain and any of the other symptoms which are typically associated with nerve problems, such as tingling, numbness and so on. Where the rupture is caused by degeneration of the disc, however, there may be no leg pain, but severe back pain will typically develop.

Ruptured discs, like bulging and herniated discs, can occur in any part of the spine but, in common with these other types, they tend to affect the lower back and neck areas most frequently. Again, the wear and tear that comes with age is significant in terms of the cause, but discs can also rupture as a result of trauma to the spine.

Quite often, the pain associated with ruptured discs will clear up of its own accord over the course of a week to ten days as the disc shrinks and inflammation of the nerve begins to settle down. In some cases, however, either the initial pain is too much for the individual to bear and so medical help needs to be sought immediately, or the pain does not abate on its own over time. Clearly, if there is any accompanying loss of bladder or bowel control, sensation of numbness in the genital area or progressive numbness or weakness of the legs, then emergency diagnosis and treatment will be required, but otherwise doctors are more likely to begin with conservative treatments and only progress to surgical procedures if absolutely necessary.

As is the case with bulging and herniated discs, the programme of treatment for a ruptured disc might include recommendation for rest (and possibly bed rest) and the limitation of activity, medication for pain relief and either medication or injections to help reduce any inflammation, as well as physical therapy and gentle exercise. Because every patient responds differently to different types of treatment regimes though, these naturally need to be tailored to the individual's specific needs and tolerances.

In those cases where pressure on the spinal nerve is evident and surgery is ultimately required, a discectomy may be performed to remove any fragments of disc which are applying pressure to the nerve or directly to the spinal cord itself. Where the entire disc needs to be removed, modern day surgical techniques now allow for an artificial disc to be inserted in place of the damaged one. These types of operations are not required, however, in the vast majority of cases.

Although a ruptured disc can cause immense amounts of pain, the prognosis for in cases is good and, in the hands of an appropriate specialist in neck and back pain, an appropriate conservative treatment course should be all that is required.

Sciatica

The term 'sciatica' is used to describe any pain caused by the irritation or compression of the sciatic nerve and, in this respect, it is actually a symptom of an underlying cause rather than strictly speaking being a condition in its own right.

The sciatic nerve extends from the lower back, through the buttocks and down the legs, stopping just below the knee, and it is the longest and widest nerve in the entire human body. Anything which irritates or compresses this nerve will basically cause mild to severe pain in the back and into the legs, but one of the most common causes is a herniated or 'slipped' disc. In addition, however, anything from strains or sprains as a result of accidents, infections within the spine, spinal stenosis (which causes compression of the sciatic nerve) and spondylolisthesis (which effectively causes the sciatic nerve to become pinched) to the more serious tumours which compress the root of the nerve and cauda equina syndrome can be the ultimate cause of sciatic pain. Even pressure on the sciatic nerve from the head of the foetus during pregnancy can lead to sciatica.

Pain from the sciatic nerve is typically only felt in one leg and it might affect anywhere from the buttock right down to the foot. Although it is often accompanied by lower back pain, the latter is generally much less severe than that which is experienced in the leg. Sometimes pain will also be accompanied by tingling, numbness or muscle weakness and in some cases it may be felt persistently, whereas in others it may be spasmodic.

Because sciatica is a symptom of an underlying problem which starts from the lower back, treatment will obviously vary according to the physician's diagnosis of that condition.

Scoliosis

So far I have mentioned a number of different conditions involving an abnormal curvature of the spine, but in each of these cases the exaggerated curve has been in a forwards or backwards direction. Scoliosis, on the other hand, is a condition in which an individual's spine is curved from side to side. Normally, when viewed from the rear on an x-ray, the spine would look straight, but in the case of somebody with scoliosis, it would be in the shape of a 'C' if there were a single curvature or an 'S' if there were a double curvature. In addition to the curve itself, the spinal column may also be twisted, which can have the effect of pulling the ribcage out of position if the problem is higher up the spine.

Scoliosis is believed to be surprisingly common, with the UK Scoliosis Association reporting that three to four children in every 1,000 require specialist supervision for the condition. It is not, however, a condition which only affects children, and in fact scoliosis can occur at any age and an estimated 20 million individuals in the USA are believed to be affected by it.

Although it sounds as though it ought to be an extremely painful condition for anyone who experiences it, in fact many people with scoliosis feel no pain or discomfort at all. There are, however, some types of scoliosis which can cause back pain, and of course the degree of the curvature will affect the nature and extent of any symptoms. To follow, you will find information concerning the five main types of scoliosis.

Idiopathic scoliosis

Most cases of scoliosis fall within the category of idiopathic scoliosis, which basically means that there is no known cause for the condition. Unlike congenital scoliosis, there is no defect in the formation of the spinal column prior to birth, although the condition may develop very shortly after birth. Interestingly though, some reports do suggest that this type of scoliosis often runs in families, with suggestions that as many as 30% of sufferers have one or more close family members suffering from the same condition.

Idiopathic scoliosis is normally classified as either early onset or late onset and both can affect boys and girls. Early onset idiopathic scoliosis is diagnosed any time between birth and the age of 10, with slightly more boys being affected in the younger age group and slightly more girls in the upper age category. In the younger age group, the spine often curves to the left, whereas in the older age category right-sided curves are more common. Although, in some cases, the curvature will resolve itself without any kind of medical intervention, conditions which are progressive do require intensive treatment to prevent further deterioration. Generally, the earlier the condition starts and the higher up the back the curve, the more pronounced the curvature and the more restricted the patient's movement.

Late onset idiopathic scoliosis is that which is diagnosed in patients who are between the ages of 10 and 18 and this is the commonest type of the condition to appear in adolescents. In fact, it is often referred to as AIS, short for adolescent idiopathic scoliosis. Once again, no cause for the condition has as yet been identified, but accurate methods to determine the risk of the curve becoming progressively worse have been developed, as well as effective methods of treatment.

Despite the fact that both early and late onset idiopathic scoliosis are fairly common, many individuals are not even aware that they have the condition and no treatment is required. Quite often, it will be parents who are alerted by a certain unevenness about the waist or shoulders, prominent shoulder blades, elevated hips or a leaning to one side, rather than the child him or herself spotting that there is something wrong. Where it is detected, however, monitoring is important to assess whether the curve is worsening, particularly because as this happens, the spinal column tends to rotate, which in turn causes the ribcage to rotate, reducing the size of the lung cavity and interfering with the ability to breathe properly. Only when the curve becomes severe (more than 60 degrees), however, is this normally a problem, but pain in the back, limbs or abdomen are all more likely as the condition progresses.

In some cases, a brace or plaster cast may be used to slow down or halt the progression of scoliosis. Only in more serious cases where the patient is actually suffering or becoming likely to suffer adverse effects, or where the curve is becoming progressively worse, would surgery be likely to become a possibility. If it were to be considered though, clearly the age of the child, as well as the size and position of the curve and the physical appearance of the individual would all be taken into account.

Aside from any pain or discomfort experienced with scoliosis, for many adolescents in particular, it is the effects of the condition on their body image which can be devastating, and it is therefore not uncommon for sufferers to experience low levels of confidence and self-esteem. In the vast majority of cases, however, those with the condition do lead full and productive lives.

Syndromic scoliosis

The term 'syndromic scoliosis' comes from the word 'syndrome' and refers to a type of the condition which occurs as part of another recognised disorder, such as the genetic disorder of the connective tissue which is known as Marfan's syndrome. Basically, people who suffer from this and certain other types of disorder are more likely to develop scoliosis and so they would normally be monitored for any signs of spinal curvature from the time that they were diagnosed with the original disorder. As is the case with idiopathic scoliosis, the condition normally becomes evident in the patient's early years.

Because syndromic scoliosis goes hand in hand with another condition, obviously there may be other health considerations which need to be taken into account when considering treatment. Generally, however, treatment would be similar to that used in the case of idiopathic scoliosis, if indeed it is required at all. In conditions which involve progressive neurological changes, however, even after surgery is performed to correct the curve, there is still the possibility that a further curvature could develop.

Degenerative scoliosis

Unlike idiopathic and syndromic scoliosis, both of which develop during an individual's early life, the degenerative form of the condition occurs in adults. In most cases, it is those who are over the age of 40 who are affected in the lumbar region of the spine. In some cases, the patient may have been diagnosed with scoliosis during childhood but the condition did not progress until middle age, whereas in others there may have been no evidence of the condition until later life. Arthritis or other conditions which cause degeneration and the uneven collapse of the intervertebral discs and facet joints and the slippage of vertebrae are, however, believed to be largely responsible for the occurrence or the reappearance of scoliosis in those who are older.

The term 'degenerative scoliosis' does not only come from the fact that the condition is the result of deterioration in the spine, but also from the fact that the spinal curvature becomes progressively worse as time goes by. Particularly where the patient is suffering from osteoporosis, the spinal curve can progress by as much as several degrees per year, thereby creating the risk of vertebral collapse.

Whereas idiopathic and syndromic scoliosis often do not present with pain or other types of symptom, the degenerative form of the condition typically does. Constant back pain is commonly experienced, as is inflammation of the vertebrae. In more severe cases, where the ribcage becomes compressed as the result of the distortion and twisting of the spine, this can cause breathing difficulties and injury to the heart and lungs, as well as leading to a greater susceptibility to chest infections such as pneumonia. In pregnant women, the additional load can put additional pressure on a spine which is already compromised.

In terms of treatment, of course much will depend on the extent and the speed of the degeneration, as well as on the severity of the symptoms. In less severe cases, conservative treatment programmes which include pain relief and anti-inflammatory medications, including epidural or facet injections, physical therapy, chiropractic or osteopathic manipulation and a weight loss regime, if necessary, are likely to be prescribed. The wearing of a back brace may also be recommended, but as the curvatures which are found in adults tend to be somewhat stiffer than those in children, correction of the curve is not likely to be as good and the aim of the brace is more about eliminating motion in the back and relieving stress on the facet joints. Where surgery is considered as an option, this is usually aimed at eliminating pain rather than addressing the curvature itself, although in some cases it can result in some improvement to the shape of the spine.

Without treatment, degenerative scoliosis can ultimately lead to physical disability which may prevent the sufferer from working and otherwise impair his or her quality of life. If managed using conservative treatments or surgical treatment where necessary, however, there is usually no reason why the individual should not be able to live a pain-free and relatively normal existence.

Neuromuscular scoliosis

Like syndromic scoliosis, neuromuscular scoliosis is a form of the condition which is linked to other illnesses or disorders. In this case though, the primary disorder is one which affects the neurological system, such as spina bifida, cerebral palsy and muscular dystrophy. Injuries to the spinal cord can also lead to the development of neuromuscular scoliosis.

What most of the underlying conditions found in neuromuscular scoliosis have in common is that they typically involve a weakness in the trunk. Either the nerves from the brain down to the spinal cord are affected or the muscles in the torso do not function properly, making it impossible for the patient to maintain an upright position and so the spine begins to curve. The slouched position that they are forced to adopt often means that kyphosis can develop, and sometimes this is in addition to a long C-shaped sideways curvature.

As many of the neurological disorders which lead to neuromuscular scoliosis are either present from birth or affect children from an early age, there is nearly always the issue of growth spurts to contend with. In those with scoliosis, these perfectly normal accelerations in developmental growth have the effect of increasing the rate of progression of the curvature and, especially for those children who are confined to a wheelchair, progressive curves can make even sitting extremely uncomfortable. In addition, as the curve becomes larger, the lung cavity decreases in size which in turn leads to shortness of breath and recurrent pneumonia.

Treatment of neuromuscular scoliosis needs to take a multidisciplinary approach which not only involves an expert in neck and back disorders, but also a neurologist who is an authority on the underlying neurological disorder. Although the use of a back brace may be recommended to help support the trunk of the patient while he or she is in a seated position, it is typically ineffective in halting the progression of the curve and so surgical treatment in the form of a long fusion tends to be the more appropriate solution. As many of these cases involve children who are quite severely disabled, however, it is essential that each case is dealt with on an individual basis and the best way forward determined in relation to the individual's current quality of life and the potential for its improvement.

Congenital scoliosis

Congenital scoliosis, as the name suggests, is caused by a developmental defect in the formation of the spinal column prior to birth, although there is little evidence to suggest that it is a hereditary condition. The abnormality usually occurs within the first six weeks of the formation of the embryo and either results in parts of vertebrae being missing or vertebrae being fused together on one side so that the spine becomes curved. As the kidneys and the heart are also formed at this stage of development, children who are born with congenital scoliosis have an increased chance of being born with abnormalities of the uro-logical and cardiac systems. In a small percentage of cases, problems with the lungs and the oesophagus may also be present.

In mild to moderate cases, scoliosis is not painful and indeed con-genital scoliosis, although it usually becomes obvious by the time the child reaches adolescence, may not be detected before then. As with the idiopathic form of the condition, it is often ill-fitting clothes, a prominent shoulder blade or uneven shoulders that give the first hint of congenital scoliosis, rather than because the child is in any pain. If the curvature is progressive, however, and becomes severe, then this puts pressure on muscles, ligaments, joints, discs and nerves, which can, of course, result in back pain and, where the nerves or spinal cord are directly affected, in weakness, numbness or a loss of co-ordination.

Monitoring of the progression of the spinal curve is very important in congenital scoliosis, particularly up to the age of five and during adolescence when growth is much more rapid. In some cases where the condition is identified early, the decision may be made to operate straight away so that a positive effect on the growth of the spine can be achieved. The operation, however, is a complex one and so needs to be given careful consideration.

Even when the curvature only appears slight when first diagnosed and any progression seems to be slow, often it can get bigger as the spine grows and of course with so much more growing to do, the likelihood is that in younger children it will worsen. Having said this, children who suffer from congenital scoliosis are normally able to participate actively in most sports and hobbies without there being any risk of the curve becoming progressively worse. In fact, as with any form of scoliosis, keeping fit and flexible by doing regular exercise such as walking, swimming, Pilates and yoga is key to living normally with the condition.

Although braces or casts can be very effective in correcting the curvature which is produced by some types of scoliosis, the congenital form is not one of these. In some cases, however, they may be recom-mended to control any compensatory curves which appear in areas of the spine where the vertebrae are normal in terms of shape and con-struction. Unless surgery is recommended, therefore, the normal treatment programme would be aimed at providing symptomatic relief via traditional medications or complementary therapies such as hydrotherapy or gentle massage, and addressing the imbalances in the muscles around the spine.

~

Scoliosis, despite sounding like a particularly frightening condition, rarely has an adverse impact on the sufferer's life. As I have said, in many cases patients experience no pain or other symptoms and there is no reason whatsoever why, from a physical perspective, they should not be able to enjoy a perfectly normal quality of life. Where children are concerned, however, and young adults in particular, the condition can cause distress if the spinal curvature becomes severe and their physical appearance is noticeably affected. It is always advisable, there-fore, to seek early diagnosis if the condition is suspected, so that treatment is not compromised by beginning once the curvature has already become severe.

Shingles

Shingles is the commonest viral infection to cause lower back pain and occurs in people who have had chickenpox at some time in the past. Once an individual has contracted the chickenpox virus, known as varicella-zoster or Herpes varicellae, basically it travels from the skin to the roots of the nerves next to the spinal cord where it lies dormant, sometimes without ever causing any further problems. In some cases, however, the virus is reactivated, causing it to travel back to the skin where it causes a rash to the area supplied by the affected nerve.

Although it is not known for certain what causes this reactivation, it may be linked to changes in the immune system, such as when there is an infection elsewhere in the body or even as a result of the natural ageing of the immune system as we grow older. Periods of stress or other types of illness may also be responsible. Generally though, greater numbers of people over the age of 50 tend to be affected, although it can appear in younger individuals, especially those whose immune system is weakened.

Shingles is a common infection, affecting one in every four or five adults. It has no gender preference and so both men and women are equally affected and suffer the same range of symptoms. The first sign that a reactivation of the virus is occurring is usually a burning sensation, shooting pain, tingling or itching along the affected nerve paths. As these typically form semi-circles around the body, it is usually just one side of the body or face which is affected, such as from the middle of the back and around to one side of the chest.

Within a few days of these early symptoms, a rash of small fluid-filled blisters appears in the same area against a background of red, swollen skin, and these will normally feel itchy and produce a burning sensation. After a further three to five days, the blisters start to burst and turn into sores which eventually scab over and heal within two to three weeks. As the blisters are filled with the chickenpox virus, this means that anyone with shingles can give chickenpox to someone who has not already had it. It is not possible, however, for one person to catch shingles from another, or for shingles to be contracted from someone with chickenpox.

An entire episode of shingles normally lasts for two to four weeks and it is not uncommon for fever or enlarged nymph nodes to accompany the shingles rash, leaving the person feeling quite unwell. Once the rash has completely disappeared, most people will return to normal and never experience the infection again. In around one in every 50 cases, however, the infection does return at least once during the remainder of the individual's lifetime. In addition, some people will experience a complication of shingles which is known as post-herpetic neuralgia.

Post-herpetic neuralgia is nerve pain in the area of a shingles rash which remains even after the rash itself has disappeared. It is believed to affect up to 25% of shingles sufferers over the age of 60, causing what can be debilitating pain for weeks, months or even years. This complication of shingles tends to be more common in older people, as well as in those who experience a particularly bad bout of the infection and, in cases where the period of pain is prolonged, it is not unusual for patients to become quite severely depressed.

Although some people who experience shingles only have the rash and no pain, for a great many others it is an extremely painful condition and so its treatment is aimed at easing pain and discomfort, as well as reducing the risk of post-herpetic neuralgia. Ordinary painkillers such as paracetamol or anti-inflammatory medications such as ibuprofen may be sufficient to relieve pain, but in other cases stronger painkillers may be required. Calamine lotion, meanwhile, can be helpful to reduce the itchiness of the rash.

Antiviral drugs (which do not actually kill the virus but stop it from multiplying) are also commonly prescribed for cases of shingles to try and limit the severity of the infection. Although there is some debate as to how effective these are in all cases, many doctors believe that they can help to prevent the occurrence of post-herpetic neuralgia. Steroids may also be recommended to reduce inflammation.

Rather than being prescribed for their more obvious purposes, tricyclic antidepressants and anticonvulsant drugs often form part of the treatment for shingles and post-herpetic neuralgia because both of these groups of drugs can be very effective at easing nerve pain. Capsaicin cream, which is often used in the treatment of arthritis and muscle, joint or nerve pain, can also be used to control pain symptoms. Capsaicin is actually the active component of chilli peppers and it works by interfering with the chemical which transmits pain impulses to the brain. Local anaesthetics applied directly to the skin, such as lidocaine plasters, can also provide relief.

Treatment of post-herpetic neuralgia can be a complex matter, not least because many of the medications, including tricyclic antidepressants and capsaicin, can cause side effects. It is important, therefore, for professional treatment to be sought and for treatment regimes to be tailored to the individual.

Spinal infections

Spinal infections, although thankfully uncommon, can be extremely dangerous, with the potential to lead to instability of the spine, neurological damage and even death. With the main symptom of the infection typically being back pain which could be attributable to any number of other causes, there is an added risk of a delay in diagnosis which allows the infection to take a firmer hold.

Spinal infections most commonly occur when another infection spreads from a different part of the body through the bloodstream, and those which originate from the urinary tract or from a wound are some of the most frequent sources. Despite the many precautions taken in hospitals to avoid surgical patients contracting an infection, some sources estimate that up to 4% of those who undergo operations develop an infection from surgical instruments or as a result of long surgeries and re-operations. The risks in terms of the latter are particularly significant in cases where a number of operations need to be carried out in the same area of the body, and generally infections which develop during a post-operative period will show themselves anywhere between three days and three months after the surgery has been carried out. Others who are in the higher risk category for contracting spinal infections are people:

- who are chronically ill, e.g. with cancer;
- whose immune system is suppressed due to human immunodeficiency virus (HIV) or acquired immunodeficiency syndrome (AIDS) or as a result of medical treatment such as for tumours;
- who are sufferers of diabetes;
- who have undergone transplant surgery;
- who are drug addicts, and particularly those who use drugs intravenously;
- who are malnourished;
- who are elderly;
- who are obese;
- who are smokers.

Spinal infections may be caused by bacteria or fungal organisms and they can affect the vertebrae which make up the spinal column (vertebral osteomyelitis), the intervertebral discs (discitis) or the tissue which surrounds the spinal cord and nerve root (epidural abscess). In some other cases it might be the space around the spinal cord which is compromised. Generally the infection will only affect one of these areas, but this is not always the case. Where it does spread to two or more areas, clearly the patient would exhibit symptoms of serious illness and the prognosis would be far less favourable.

The symptoms of a spinal infection can vary in intensity and in some cases may only be quite mild. Generally though, they would include some or all of the following:

- fever;
- chills;
- headaches;
- stiffness in the neck;
- pain which is often unrelenting;
- redness and tenderness of a wound;
- wound drainage which could vary in colour;
- fatigue;
- loss of appetite;
- weakness, tingling or numbness in the arms and/or legs.

The following is a more detailed description of each of the different types of spinal infection, along with the specific causes, symptoms, treatments and prognosis for each.

Vertebral osteomyelitis

Vertebral osteomyelitis is an infection in the large, cylindrical part of the vertebra which is known as the vertebral body. Although the infection can be caused by bacteria or fungus, it is the bacterial or pyogenic form which is commoner and the organism which is most frequently responsible is *Staphylococcus aureus*. It can affect the lumbar, thoracic or cervical region of the spine, but reports suggest that the latter cases account for only between 3 and 6% of the total. In cases where vertebral osteomyelitis does occur in the neck region, however, the risk of serious neurological damage and paralysis is much higher than if it occurs in either of the other two regions.

The infection which causes vertebral osteomyelitis can spread to a bone in a number of ways. It can, for example, begin from skin, muscles or tendons or pass to the bone through the blood. It can also start after an individual has undergone bone surgery, especially if the operation was as the result of an injury which required metal rods or plates to be inserted into the bone. Whereas in younger patients it is more likely to be the long bones such as the femur which are affected, in adults it is more commonly the hips, feet and vertebrae. Because the spleen, which is part of the lymphatic system, plays a key role in fighting infection, patients who have their spleen removed are also at higher risk of contracting vertebral osteomyelitis.

Bone pain is one of the key symptoms of this type of infection, as are localised swelling and redness and fever. Pain may also be experienced in the lower back, and there may be swelling in the ankles, feet and legs as well as chills, excessive sweating, weight loss and, in cases where there is a wound or incision from an earlier surgery, drainage. Symptoms often build up over time and it can take a period of 8–12 weeks before a firm diagnosis is made. The back pain, which is typically the first sign of the infection, starts off at a low level and is localised, but as time goes on it becomes increasingly severe, to the extent where even complete bed rest does not help to relieve it. If the infection continues untreated, it can lead to the destruction and collapse of the vertebral body.

As you might expect with an infection, antibiotics are essential in killing off the bacteria and limiting the amount of damage to the bone and the surrounding tissues, and these are often given intravenously to achieve a more rapid effect. In some cases, a cocktail of different antibiotics might be used to attack different types of bacteria, but whichever types of drugs are prescribed, they will generally be given intravenously for a period of at least 4–6 weeks, and may be followed up by a further six-week course of tablets to be taken orally.

Although most cases of acute vertebral osteomyelitis can be treated successfully using conservative methods, in cases where the destruction of the vertebra is ongoing or the infection does not appear to be going away, surgery may be required to remove any dead bone tissue and/or any metal rods or plates which are close to the site of the infection. Several complications of acute osteomyelitis can, however, occur, even after surgery has been carried out. Either pus which is produced in the bone can result in an abscess which effectively deprives the bone of its blood supply, or the infection can spread into surrounding tissues or the bloodstream, causing symptoms which can come and go for prolonged periods of time and turning the condition into one which is chronic.

As with any other type of infection, treating vertebral osteomyelitis as early as possible is desirable and it is especially important for those in one of the higher risk categories to seek medical attention promptly, should they develop any signs of the infection.

Discitis

Discitis, or disc space infection, is the name which is given to swelling and irritation of the intervertebral disc caused by a bacterial or viral infection or, in some cases, by autoimmune diseases in which the immune system attacks healthy cells in the body by mistake. Although the name suggests that the disc is the source of the infection, some believe that it stems from infection of the vertebral end plates (the top and bottom parts of the vertebral bodies which interface with the discs), while others contend that the infection travels from another part of the body altogether. In many cases, the infection has been known to develop after an invasive procedure such as a lumbar puncture, and this is thought to be because microorganisms are introduced into the body as the procedure is carried out and these in turn lead to infection. As with vertebral osteomyelitis, the offending organism often turns out to be *Staphylococcus aureus*. Severe trauma to the back can also be the primary cause of the inflammation.

Discitis is not a common condition, but when it does occur it tends to affect more children than adults. Rarely is it found in elderly people because the discs naturally become smaller and less spongy with age and so are less prone to inflammation. It can affect the cervical spine, but is more often found in the discs in the thoracic or lumbar regions. Usually discitis only affects a single disc, but in some cases it can spread to adjacent ones.

The symptoms of discitis are typically subtle to begin with but get gradually worse, and the infection is characterised by:

- progressively worsening back pain;
- difficulty in rising from a seated position and standing;
- abdominal pain;
- stiffness of the back;
- tenderness around the spine;
- increased curvature of the back.

Unlike vertebral osteomyelitis, discitis does not present with symptoms affecting the entire bodily system and so it would be unusual for the infection to be accompanied by, for example, a high temperature. In children particularly, however, the severe pain associated with the condition can lead to irritability and in some cases youngsters may refuse to sit up, stand or walk in order to avoid flexing the spine.

Often when x-rays of the spine are carried out in cases of discitis, they reveal a narrowing of the disc space, as well as some erosion of the vertebral end plates. Treatment typically consists of bed rest, and sometimes in the case of young children plaster cast immobilisation, along with the prescription of pain relief and anti-inflammatory medications. Antibiotics are also used to treat the underlying cause of the infection and, if the condition does not improve with these alone, steroids may be administered. These conservative forms of treatment are, in the vast majority of cases, highly effective, and it is extremely rare for the condition to lead to chronic back pain once treatment has been sought. The rare exception to this might occur where the discitis was caused by an autoimmune disease, as often such diseases are long-term illnesses which present ongoing problems.

Spinal epidural abscess

A spinal epidural abscess is basically an accumulation of infected material or pus which forms in the space around the dura, the outer covering of the spinal cord and nerve root. Usually they occur in the upper or lower back regions and often there is an underlying infection present, although this may have originated from a completely different area of the body. A dental abscess, for example, could potentially cause the spread of infection which leads to a spinal epidural abscess.

Epidural abscesses of the spinal column are rare, but they can be extremely serious and even fatal if left undiagnosed and untreated. The infected material can surround the spinal cord and/or the nerve roots, generating sufficient pressure to affect the body's neurological function and ultimately causing paralysis. In addition, the infection itself can cause inflammation and swelling which also compresses the spinal cord.

The infection which leads to a spinal epidural abscess is usually caused by *Staphylococcus aureus* or *Escherichia coli*, although in some cases it may be a fungus that is responsible. Those who are at greatest risk are people who have undergone invasive procedures involving the spine or back surgery, those who have infections of the bloodstream, people who frequently experience boils (especially on the back or scalp) and those with vertebral osteomyelitis. Those who engage in intravenous drug use are also at increased risk, as are those who have experienced even minor back injuries or trauma. In the case of post-operative infections, smokers are in a group which is considered to be very high-risk.

The symptoms of a spinal epidural abscess can be quite subtle and limited to a sensation not dissimilar to pins and needles or a feeling of mild weakness. Backache in the lower part of the back, however, is quite common, and often this starts off as mild but slowly gets worse. The pain might move to the hips, legs or feet or spread into the shoulder, arm or hand. Chills and fever might also accompany the pain sensations in the earlier stages of the condition.

As the compression of the spinal nerve roots or spinal cord becomes more intense, the individual might experience loss of movement in a particular area of the body, numbness, weakness, paralysis and/or the loss of bladder or bowel control, as well as severe back pain. The severity of these symptoms will depend upon where on the spine the abscess is located and the extent to which the nerve root or the spinal cord is compressed, but if any of these latter symptoms are experienced it is important to seek medical advice as a matter of urgency.

In very serious cases, surgical intervention may be necessary to decompress the spinal cord before permanent paralysis results, and this is normally achieved by a procedure known as a laminectomy which involves draining the abscess. Where it is not possible to drain the abscess entirely, the laminectomy would be followed up by the same conservative treatments which are used in cases where the abscess is detected earlier, including intravenous administration of what may be a combination of antibiotics and medication to reduce inflammation and swelling, as well as that to relieve pain.

The prognosis for spinal epidural abscesses is variable and normally depends upon how quickly it is detected and treated. In the worst case scenario where the condition remains untreated, spinal cord compression can be so great that it causes severe and permanent paralysis and even death. In other cases, injury to the spinal cord which is caused by the pressure of the abscess can lead to chronic back pain which requires long-term pain management, and an abscess which is not drained completely may return or cause scarring of the spinal cord. If caught and treated early, however, the prognosis is good and some people make a complete recovery.

If a spinal epidural abscess is suspected, it is vital to seek urgent medical attention by attending the emergency room at the nearest hospital or calling the emergency services.

Spinal stenosis

The word 'stenosis' comes from the Ancient Greek for 'narrowing' and in spinal stenosis it is the spinal canal which narrows. The spinal canal, or vertebral canal as it is also known, is the space in the vertebrae through which the spinal cord passes, and basically it acts as protection for the cord and the spinal nerve roots. In spinal stenosis, excessive bone growth, the thickening of tissues such as ligaments and cartilage, or bulging or herniated intervertebral discs can cause this space to become narrower so that the spinal cord and nerve roots are squeezed or irritated.

Both men and women are affected by spinal stenosis, but the condition is far more common in those over the age of 50, as the process which causes the spinal canal to narrow is mostly age-related. As we grow older, the ligaments which connect the tissues in between the bones of the spine naturally thicken, and the intervertebral discs start to show signs of wear and tear and lose their ability to absorb shock in the same way that they did when we were younger. The facet joints too may begin to degenerate and, in those who suffer from degenerative arthritis, small bone spurs might develop, all of which can contribute to the narrowing of the spinal canal. In addition, genetic factors, smoking, traumatic injuries, anything which affects the blood flow to the lumbar spine or being in a job which involves a great deal of heavy lifting can accelerate degeneration so that younger people may also be affected.

Spinal stenosis can affect the cervical, thoracic or lumbar region of the spine, but in most people it is the lumbar region or lower back which is compromised. Although many people do not suffer any symptoms at all from this process of normal wear and tear, for others it can cause pain which might vary from dull to severe and affect the lower back or the buttocks, particularly when the person is standing or walking. Weakness in the legs or a feeling that the legs are tired is common too, and some may experience numbness, tingling or feelings of hot or cold in the legs, symptoms which can lead to a certain clumsiness and frequent falls. Often, sufferers find that they experience relief from much of their discomfort by sitting, lying down and particularly by bending forwards from the waist as this effectively enlarges the space available for the nerves. Walking on the flat or downhill, standing straight or leaning backwards on the other hand, tend to increase the levels of pain.

Where stenosis affects the neck area, pain, stiffness, numbness and weakness in the neck, shoulders, arms and legs are the most typical symptoms. Clumsiness of the hands may be experienced too, along with tingling, pins and needles or burning sensations in whichever extremity is affected. As with stenosis which affects the back, if cervical stenosis becomes severe, there can also be a loss of bladder or bowel control and, in rare but severe cases where the problem occurs in the neck, there can be a resulting loss of function or even paralysis. Cervical stenosis is quite often related to some kind of injury or trauma to the neck, such as a whiplash injury, although the symptoms of the condition may not become evident until many months or even years after the accident.

The symptoms of spinal stenosis are normally controlled using conservative treatments, with surgery to relieve the pressure on the nerves only being considered if the symptoms are severe, worsen considerably or begin to affect normal daily activities. Pain relief medication, anti-inflammatory drugs and/or muscle relaxants may be prescribed, but physical therapy and exercise are also important parts of treatment and help to strengthen muscles and improve flexibility. Aerobic activity such as cycling has been shown to be beneficial and, where excess weight is putting an extra load on the spine, a weight loss diet may be recommended. In certain cases, corticosteroid injections may also be used to help reduce nerve inflammation.

For many people, the symptoms of spinal stenosis can have quite a considerable effect on their daily lives and, because walking and standing often cause intense pain, there is the danger that they might confine themselves to their homes and become increasingly isolated. Seeking the help of a reputable pain management consultant is therefore very important in terms of restoring a good quality of life.

Spinal syringomyelia

Often caused by trauma to the spinal cord such as might result from a car accident or a serious fall, or congenital developmental problems such as Chiari I malformation, spinal syringomyelia is a condition in which a cyst (called a syrinx) or a collection of fluid forms within the spinal cord itself. Where compression of the spinal cord is the cause of the disorder, a herniated disc, severe spinal stenosis, instability of the spine or tumours may be responsible. As with stenosis, if a motoring accident or fall was what contributed to the condition, syringomyelia may lie dormant and not manifest itself until many years later when troublesome symptoms eventually warrant medical attention.

The spinal cord, of course, is what connects the brain to the nerves in the extremities and so those with the condition are not only likely to experience pain and stiffness in the back, shoulders, arms or legs, but also weakness and numbness in the arms, hands and legs which can cause difficulties with holding objects, writing and raising the arms, as well as problems with balance and gait. In addition, the sufferer may experience headaches, disruption to body temperature and the loss of the ability to feel extremes of hot and cold. Bladder and bowel control and sexual function can also be affected. Usually, symptoms become progressively worse over a period of years and often the condition is not diagnosed until the sufferer reaches middle age.

Magnetic resonance imaging (MRI) scans are the main tools used for diagnosing syringomyelia and not only do the fluid collections which characterise the disorder show up very clearly on these, but also any tumours which might be present. In cases where the condition presents without symptoms or in those where symptoms are not progressing, syringomyelia will not normally be treated, although sufferers will generally be advised to avoid any activities which involve straining. If symptoms do exist but the condition is not sufficiently advanced to warrant surgery, then treatment is aimed solely at pain management as drugs have no curative effect on the disorder.

Typically, where pain is severe, more than one type of pain medication will be prescribed to deal with what might be described as 'classic' back pain and neuropathic pain which comes from the nerves and usually exhibits as shooting or stabbing pains. Over-the-counter analgesics such as paracetamol, meanwhile, would be used to combat headaches. In chronic cases where medication is used on a long-term basis, monitoring with blood tests is important in order to assess whether there are any adverse effects on the liver, and periodic MRI scans should also be carried out to detect any progression of the condition.

Where syringomyelia is more severe, the only viable treatment is via surgery. As draining the syrinx does not necessarily eliminate the symptoms and can sometimes cause more problems than it solves because it involves making an incision in the spinal cord itself, the aim of surgery is to address the condition which allowed the cyst to form in the first place. Where Chiari I malformation is the underlying condition, the operation is designed to make more space for the cerebellum (which plays an important role in voluntary motor movement, balance and muscle tone) at the base of the skull and the upper part of the cervical spine without entering the brain or spinal cord. In the case of a herniated disc, the procedure would be a discectomy to remove a fragment of the disc, and in cases involving spinal instability, fusion of the affected vertebrae would be recommended. Because spinal surgery carries with it certain risks, however, the benefits of operating need to be carefully weighed against any potential complications.

Sometimes, even after surgery to address the root cause, the syrinx still persists, in which case a shunt (a system comprising a plastic catheter, drainage tubes and valves which drains the fluid into a cavity such as the abdomen) may be inserted to stop the progression of symptoms and provide relief from pain, headaches and tightness. In addition to the fact that a shunt may not necessarily work for all patients, its use also carries risks, such as of damage to the spinal cord, infection, blockage or haemorrhage, and so this too needs to be discussed fully with an expert physician.

Spinal tumours

Spinal tumours are probably the greatest fear of anyone who suffers from neck or back pain, but in fact only in a very small percentage of cases are tumours of any type responsible for the symptoms. In the UK, it is estimated that 750 cases of primary spinal tumours are diagnosed each year.

Spinal tumours can either arise directly from the structures of the spine, in which case they are known as primary tumours, or they can spread to the spine from elsewhere in the body and are known as secondary tumours or metastases. In some cases, there may be more than one secondary spinal tumour. Primary tumours are much rarer and those which develop as a result of secondary deposits of cancer most commonly spread from the lung, breast, prostate or bowel. Whether primary or secondary, they can develop at any point along the spine, from the top of the neck down to the sacrum (the large triangular bone at the base of the spine) and tumours of the bone are the most common type, although these are nearly always secondaries. Bone tumours can destroy the bone and cause spinal deformity.

In some cases spinal tumours grow in between the dura (the protective membrane which surrounds the spinal cord) and the spinal canal (extradural), whilst in others they appear inside the dura, within the spinal canal but not within the nerves (intradural). Very occasionally, the tumour might grow inside the spinal canal and within the nerves (intramedullary), although this is more common in the cervical region of the spine.

As is the case with tumours which develop elsewhere in the body, spinal tumours can either be benign (non-cancerous) or malignant (cancerous). Those which are benign are usually intradural and rarely grow in the bones of the spine. Even though these types of tumour in themselves do not normally compromise the strength of the spinal column, sometimes their removal, which might be required to stop any damage or injury to the spinal cord or nerves, does.

Benign tumours can sometimes grow for many years but, because the space in the spinal canal is so limited, they rarely reach any great size before being detected. The only exception to this are those which develop in the sacrum, which may grow quite considerably before producing any noticeable symptoms. Malignant tumours, on the other hand, have a tendency to grow much more quickly, but the speed at which the symptoms develop does not necessarily correlate with the speed of the growth and does not normally determine the effectiveness of treatment.

The reasons why benign and malignant tumours develop are not known, and neither do doctors yet understand why some are cancerous and others not so, which makes determining risk factors currently impossible. What is known, however, is that nearly all spinal tumours occur randomly rather than as a result of a genetic abnormality. MRI scans and computerised tomography (CT) scans are normally used to diagnose spinal tumours, and computerised axial tomography (CAT) scans are generally used to investigate other possible tumours elsewhere in the body.

Spinal tumours, rather than just causing a single symptom, tend to generate a combination of warning signs, although even some of these may relate to other co-existing illnesses or diseases. Generally, however, the most common symptoms include pain in or near the spine, problems which affect either one limb or both legs and bladder or bowel control problems. It is important to remember though, that these symptoms could be indicative of many other conditions which are either directly or indirectly related to the back or neck.

Pain might be felt in the neck or back, may be worse at night and is not relieved by rest. Numbness, tingling or weakness can be experienced in one limb, and there may also be some pain in the limb, but again it is important to remember that herniated discs and a number of other much more common conditions can also cause the same symptoms. As we have seen, problems which affect both legs in the form of numbness, tingling or weakness and get progressively worse, or problems with bladder or bowel control are normally an indication that there is pressure on the spinal cord or the nerves in the spine and these should always be treated seriously. Whilst there is a possibility that the pressure is being caused by a spinal tumour, there are various other potential causes which need to be investigated as a matter of urgency.

In some cases where a spinal tumour is detected, it may be necessary to carry out a biopsy to establish whether it is benign or malignant, as clearly this will affect the course of treatment which is offered. Sometimes this can be done under local anaesthetic using a large needle, but where this is not possible, a small operation may be necessary. Either way, the results of the tests are normally available within a few days of the biopsy having been conducted. Once the type of tumour has been established, treatment would then be decided according to whether its aim is to reduce or alleviate pain or provide a cure and might depend greatly on the patient's life expectancy and overall state of health. Particularly in the case of malignant tumours, the options for treatment will involve a team of experts which might comprise a spine surgeon, oncologist, neuroradiologist and pain management specialist.

In cases where the objective is pain relief and preventing any further damage by the tumour or complications, a brace or corset may be recommended. The brace not only helps to stabilise the spinal column, but may also assist in reducing pain levels. Pain therapy, meanwhile, is likely to include anti-inflammatory medication and pain relief medication which may be administered orally or intravenously.

Where the aim is to achieve a cure for the tumour, the options include surgery, radiotherapy or chemotherapy. In some cases, steroids are also used at the time of surgery or during a course of radiotherapy to reduce swelling and provide some degree of protection from compression.

Surgical treatment is used to deal with benign tumours and also for some malignant types. In the case of those which are benign, it may be possible for the whole tumour to be removed but, depending upon the position of the growth, this is not always possible because of the risk of potentially serious damage to the spinal cord. Where such a risk does exist, a small part of the tumour may simply be left behind.

Tumours of the bone, although they should theoretically be easier to remove because the nerves and spinal cord are protected by the membrane which surrounds them, are not always easy to remove entirely either and much will depend on the size of the growth, its location and how easy it is to access. In addition, there is the added complication of ensuring that the stability of the spinal column is not compromised. Even if the entire growth cannot be removed, however, it is normally possible to take away enough of it to relieve any pressure on the spinal cord and nerves and so allow recovery from weakness or paralysis. In cases where the strength of the spine is compromised, there may be a need to insert an implant, which clearly extends the operating time and period of recovery.

Radiotherapy is often the treatment of choice for malignant tumours and it works by using a high energy X-ray to kill cancer cells, shrink a tumour or prevent growth. Sometimes it will be the only form of treatment, but often it is used after surgery to kill off any remaining disease. Generally, the patient would undergo multiple treatments on a daily basis to cure a tumour, but it can also be used as a single treatment to provide pain relief. Patients who undergo radiotherapy treatment sometimes experience a temporary worsening of their symptoms, as well as inflammation of the skin. Other potential side effects include changes in the bone marrow and bone fractures.

Again, chemotherapy is used to destroy the cancerous cells which make up a malignant tumour and it does this by interfering with cell growth and affecting the reproduction of cells. This form of treatment is mainly used for secondary spinal tumours and may be combined with other types of treatment. The side effects of chemotherapy drugs might include hair loss or thinning of the hair, nausea, fatigue, effects on fertility and soreness of the mouth, but most of these subside once treatment has been completed.

The prognosis for people with spinal tumours is highly variable and depends to a great degree on the nature and extent of the underlying condition and how effective the treatment has been, as well as on whether there is any degree of paralysis. Benign tumours can often be completely removed and, where there has been no long-term paralysis, complete recovery is entirely possible. In some cases, malignant primary tumours can also be completely removed, and once again there is a good chance of complete recovery with little chance of the tumour recurring.

Where the prognosis is less good is in those cases where the spinal tumour is secondary to cancer which has spread from elsewhere in the body. Much will depend on the type of cancer, the degree to which it has spread and the effectiveness of the treatment.

Regardless of whether a spinal tumour is benign or malignant, if there has been severe compression of the spinal cord and nerves resulting in complete paralysis, recovery will depend on how long the paralysis has been present. The spinal cord and nerves do not recover quickly if they have been badly damaged or compressed and the longer the paralysis has been present, the less likely it is that the patient will fully recover.

Spondylosis

Spondylosis is another term for degenerative arthritis, spinal osteoarthritis, degenerative joint disease, spinal arthritis and arthritis of the facet joints. Please refer to the section headed 'Degenerative or Osteoarthritis'.

Spondylolysis

Spondylolysis and spondylolisthesis, the latter of which is covered under the next heading, are separate but closely related conditions, with the former often occurring first.

The condition known as spondylolysis occurs when a crack forms in a specific part of the facet joint which is known as the 'pars interarticularis'. The bone, which forms part of the structure which protects the spinal cord, fractures on one or both sides and causes the vertebra to become unstable, much as would be the case if a hinge on a door became loose. Although this can happen in the thoracic vertebrae and in any of the bones which make up the lumbar spine, most often it occurs in the lowest of the lumbar vertebrae which is numbered L5.

Stress fractures are frequently the cause of spondylolysis, and frequently it is children and adolescents and those who take part in sports such as gymnastics, football, diving and martial arts who are most at risk. In children and adolescents whose spines are still developing, the pars interarticularis is the weakest and so the most vulnerable part of the vertebra, and this, combined with doing sports in which the spine is repeatedly bent backwards, accounts for why as many as 6% of children are affected by the condition. Childhood injuries, however, do not account for all cases of spondylolysis and adult sportspersons are also at risk. In some cases the condition can also be present at birth and, in adults, one of the most common causes is degenerative arthritis.

Many doctors believe that spondylolysis occurs because of a genetic weakness of the pars interarticularis and, as the condition does indeed seem to run in families and to be more prevalent in certain populations, a genetic link which perhaps causes a tendency towards thin vertebral bone certainly seems possible.

The symptoms which are fairly typical of the condition are pain and stiffness which is usually felt in the centre of the lower back. Often the pain worsens with activity and eases with rest, and bending backwards increases the intensity of the pain. Doctors refer to this type of back pain as mechanical pain, because the likelihood is that it comes from excess movement between the vertebrae. As the condition worsens, pain which radiates down one or both legs may also be experienced and this is probably due to pressure on and irritation of the nerves close to the fracture.

As with any fracture, the body tries to heal the crack in the pars interarticularis, but this process can cause extra cartilage to grow at the site of the injury. If too much cartilage builds up, then it can push into the opening where the nerves exit the spine, squeezing the nerve and causing pain and weakness in the leg and often a sensation of pins and needles.

Because the symptoms of spondylolysis often resolve themselves with rest or the wearing of a back brace, surgery is not normally necessary and conservative treatments and pain management are usually all that are required. An X-ray may also be taken every few months just to check that the area is healing as it should do. Wearing a rigid back brace or cast for several months can be useful, particularly in cases where the fracture occurred quite recently, as it stops the spine from moving and so helps the bones to knit back together properly. In addition, the lack of movement decreases the chance of inflammation and associated pain. Where pain and inflammation are issues, however, anti-inflammatory drugs and pain medications may be prescribed.

Physical therapies can also be particularly useful in treating spondylolysis, as certain exercises and postures can help greatly to ease symptoms, as well as improving the strength and control of the muscles in the back and the abdomen. Where the patient is involved in a sport which led to the injury, it can also be helpful for the therapist to observe the activity with a view to suggesting changes to technique or equipment which will improve performance and prevent future problems. Treatments of heat, cold, ultrasound and electrical stimulation may also be used to control pain and muscle spasms.

Although most cases of spondylolysis respond extremely well to these conservative treatments and a full recovery is made, if nonsurgical treatment is ineffective then surgery may be recommended. Usually this will involve a laminectomy to relieve compression of the spinal nerves or a posterior lumbar fusion in which small grafts of bone are laid over the problem area at the back of the spine. In some cases, the surgeon may also attach metal plates and screws to prevent the two vertebrae from moving, although this is usually unnecessary as in around 90% of cases involving children, the fusion is perfectly successful.

Spondylolisthesis

Spondylolisthesis often, although not always, occurs in the wake of spondylolysis. In the case of spondylolisthesis, what happens is that one vertebra slips forward in relation to the adjacent one. As I described previously, this is the precise reverse of what happens in retrolisthesis.

Like spondylolysis, spondylolisthesis can be present at birth, can result from injury or can be caused by degenerative arthritis. In adults over the age of 50, the latter is the main cause of the condition and in some cases this can also lead to spinal stenosis or narrowing of the spinal canal. In these cases, the disorder is not usually preceded by spondylolysis. Once again, there appears to be a strong possibility that spondylolisthesis may be hereditary, and indeed 30–50% of the Inuit people are reported to suffer from the disorder.

Spondylolisthesis can occur in the thoracic spine or at any level in the lumbar spine, but typically it is the lowest vertebra in the lumbar spine which is affected, with the body of the L5 vertebra slipping forward on to the upper vertebral body of the sacrum (S1). When this happens, there not only tends to be a general stiffening of the back, but the hamstrings, a group of muscles which extend down the back of the thigh to the knee, tend to tighten, bringing about changes in both posture and gait. Typically, a person suffering from the condition will look as though he or she is leaning forward slightly and, where spondylolisthesis is more advanced, the decreased mobility in the hamstrings may cause the pelvis to rotate more when walking, so giving the appearance that the individual is waddling rather than walking normally.

Although some people do not experience any symptoms with spondylolisthesis, for others it can be a very painful condition. Not only does the tightness of the hamstrings contribute to the discomfort, but pain in the lower back can often be accompanied by muscle spasms and intermittent shocks of sciatic pain which travel down through the buttock and the back of the thigh. Tingling, numbness and weakness may also be experienced if the nerves are affected, and both sitting and standing up from a seated position can be painful and difficult and it may feel as though there is a slipping sensation in the area of the injury. Because increased activity tends to cause inflammation of the soft tissues in the area of the spondylolisthesis, the days following the activity are typically filled with more intense pain which is only relieved by rest. Even bouts of coughing or sneezing can amplify the levels of pain in patients with spondylolisthesis.

Where no symptoms exist, generally there is no need to treat spondylolisthesis, although regular check-ups are advised to ensure that the condition is not progressing. Where treatment is required, this might include medication to relieve pain and reduce inflammation, physical therapies and manipulative treatments to help with pain symptoms and relieve any pressure on the nerves, and exercises which are designed to increase mobility in the lumbar spine and the hamstrings as well as to strengthen the abdominal muscles. Normally, a short period of rest during which activities such as bending and lifting are avoided will also be prescribed to help alleviate symptoms. In some cases, doctors may recommend the wearing of a back brace for a short period of time in order to immobilise the spine and aid the healing process, and this may also help to reduce pain and muscle spasms.

Where conservative treatments fail to bring about any improvement to an individual's symptoms or the vertebral slippage continues, surgery may become necessary. Generally, this would involve a spinal fusion being carried out to rejoin the lumbar spine and the sacrum and, if there is any likelihood that the slippage might recur, screws or pins may be placed across the area to hold the bone graft in place. Sometimes the vertebrae will be moved back into their normal positions before the fusion is carried out, but as this does carry a risk of injury to the nerve, often the bones are simply fused in the position where they are resting after the slip. In cases where there is evidence of compression of the nerves in the spine, surgical treatment will also address these by creating more room for the nerve roots.

The prognosis for anyone suffering from spondylolisthesis is generally very good and most people respond well to conservative treatments without requiring surgery. If severe symptoms do continue, then surgery to decompress the nerve can alleviate those in the leg, while lumbar fusion can put an end to, or at least significantly reduce back pain.

Whiplash

One of the commonest causes of neck pain is the whiplash injury which is frequently the result of road traffic accidents but can also be the result of sporting accidents, serious falls or even physical assaults. As you have no doubt seen from the many television advertisements urging drivers and passengers to wear seat belts, what happens when a car is hit from behind is that the weight of the neck, along with all eight pounds or so of the weight of the head, are propelled violently forwards and then backwards. One second, the structures of the neck are being stretched and strained, and the next they are being compressed, all of which can lead, among other things, to stretched or torn muscles and ligaments, dislocation of the bones in the neck and the compression of nerves. In many cases, it is not just a single part of the neck which is affected by the accident, but several, making diagnosis more complicated for doctors who do not specialise in these types of injuries.

Whiplash symptoms might appear immediately or within minutes or hours of the accident, and in some cases they will not occur for several days or even much later. In fact, where the individual sustains other injuries, these may heal long before the whiplash injury becomes apparent, and in cases where there are no other external injuries, often accident victims will walk away believing themselves to have come through the incident entirely unscathed.

The commonest symptoms of a whiplash injury tend to be:

- headaches;
- neck pain;
- swelling in the neck;
- stiffness or tenderness which is felt in the neck and at the back of the head;
- muscle spasms in the side or back of the neck;
- shooting pains which extend from the neck into the shoulder or arm.

Although it is always advisable to call a doctor immediately after the injury, this is especially important if the individual experiences:

- memory loss;
- periods of unconsciousness;
- severe pains in the back of the head;
- pins and needles in the shoulders and arms;
- a sensation of heaviness in the arms;
- dizziness, blurred vision, pain in the jaw, pain on swallowing or unusual sensations in the skin on the face which persist.

If a fracture or dislocation of the cervical spine is suspected, then the patient will be X-rayed, but X-rays, MRI scans and CT scans will not show up a whiplash injury and so diagnosis is usually made based on the patient's description of his or her symptoms. In less severe accidents, symptoms typically pass within a few weeks, during which time it is usually better to keep the neck active and moving. Your doctor may recommend the use of ice therapy during the first 24 hours after the accident, as well as prescribing pain and anti-inflammatory medications and/or muscle relaxants to relieve the symptoms. You may also be advised to carry out specific gentle neck exercises to help lessen any symptoms of stiffness.

Usually, the chances of making a complete recovery from a whiplash injury are very good and symptoms typically pass within a few weeks. Should pain persist for longer than four to six weeks or numbness, weakness or persistent pins and needles develop, however, it is important to seek further medical advice.

In some cases, symptoms continue long after the initial trauma and develop into what is known as whiplash syndrome. This is frequently characterised by continual pain and headaches, reduced movement at the back of the neck, pains in the lumbar region of the back, tingling in the arms, fatigue and sleep disruptions. In some cases, and particularly where the whiplash injury was severe, these symptoms can persist for months or even years and may even result in long-term problems. Reports suggest a 40% chance of experiencing symptoms after three months and an 18% chance after two years.

Because there can sometimes be quite a long period between the accident which caused the whiplash injury and the point at which the neck pain reveals itself, many people believe that it is then too late to pursue a claim against the driver who caused the accident. With proper representation and the help of a medico-legal expert, however, there is usually no reason why the claim cannot go ahead and be successful. You can find out more about the role of medico-legal experts and how they can help in pursuing such a claim in Part 4 of this book.

Limiting the risk of neck and back pain

As you can see, the causes of neck and back pain are many, but in some cases, there is little or nothing that can be done to limit the risk of suffering from neck and back problems, such as if they occur as a result of age, injury or certain medical conditions such as rheumatoid arthritis or spinal stenosis.

The natural process of ageing has much to answer for in terms of neck and back-related problems and, unfortunately, those over the age of 50 can do nothing to prevent the degeneration of the various structures of the spine which happen simply because of general wear and tear. Risk factors which can be controlled, however, include:

- poor posture;
- adopting awkward positions which put stress on the back;
- heavy physical work;
- careless lifting and bending;
- stress;

- depression;
- poor general physical condition and lack of exercise;
- drug abuse;
- smoking.

Some of these controllable risk factors are what might be described as secondary causes, which basically set up a vicious cycle of behaviour and lead to recurrent symptoms. An initial bout of pain or injury, for example, might cause a person to tense their muscles, limit their range of movement, move in particular ways to guard against pain or even become completely inactive. Although these things might appear to help at the time, however, ultimately they can cause the shortening of ligaments and the shortening and weakening of muscles which in turn not only causes more pain, but also leads to muscle spasms and fatigue.

Stress or depression which result from worrying about a neck or back problem or which stem from an impaired quality of life due to neck or back pain, can also set up the same vicious cycle. Where timely diagnosis and treatment are sought, however, there is usually no need for patients to suffer either mental or physical distress. Even in cases where the specific cause of neck or back pain cannot be determined, if there are no 'red flag' warning signs, then the condition is extremely unlikely to be dangerous and patients can save themselves any undue concern, not to mention pain and discomfort, by visiting an appropriately qualified and experienced pain management specialist.

Carers

Before I leave the subject of the causes of neck and back pain, there is one particularly important group of people that I would like to address, and that is carers. People who look after partners, family members or friends who are sick, frail or disabled are some of the most vulnerable in terms of neck and back problems as they are frequently involved in manual handling tasks. In fact, it is estimated that around half of all unpaid carers suffer from lower back pain.

While the treatments for carers are no different from those for others, it is vital that carers reduce their initial risk of injury. A good pain-management specialist should be able to provide advice on lifting techniques and posture, as well as recommending exercises which are aimed at strengthening the back muscles and keeping the spine supple and strong. In addition, St John Ambulance provides a carer support programme at various locations throughout the UK and the NHS offers information, advice and support to carers via its Carers Direct website (www.nhs.uk/carersdirect/Pages/CarersDirectHome.aspx) and confidential helpline. Numerous local support groups also exist for carers and these can be found by carrying out an internet search.

4

Diagnosing Neck and Back Problems

With so many different causes of neck and back pain, diagnosing the problem is not always a straightforward matter for doctors, and in some cases it may not be possible at all to get to the root cause. That having been said, just because the initial cause cannot be identified does not mean to say that the symptoms cannot be successfully dealt with or managed or that the condition is necessarily a serious one. In fact, more dangerous disorders such as tumours are typically far easier to pick up than injuries such as whiplash.

In order to make as complete and accurate diagnosis of the cause of neck or back pain as possible, and so be able to design an appropriate treatment programme, health care professionals rely on a combination of up to four basic things:

- a detailed patient history;
- a physical examination;
- diagnostic tests;
- laboratory tests.

In this chapter, I will look at each of these in more detail.

Patient history

As you will have seen from the previous chapter, different aspects of an individual's personal and medical history can make certain conditions which cause neck and back pain more or less likely. Some conditions, for example, are more likely to occur in younger or older age groups, while others might occur as the result of trauma or injury. Some have possible genetic links, while others might have more to do with an individual's occupation or leisure activities. The doctor's first step, therefore, is to ask a series of detailed questions which will help to rule in or out different possibilities and determine the cause of the problem.

Normally, your doctor will talk you through the questions that he or she needs to ask, but in some cases you may be requested to complete a written questionnaire initially and then follow up with further discussion. Either way, the more detailed your answers, the easier it will be for your doctor to make an accurate diagnosis. The type of questions that you are likely to be asked include:

- Where do you feel the pain?
- How severe is the pain?
- What type of pain (dull, throbbing, aching, etc.) do you experience?
- Does the pain radiate to other parts of the body?
- When did the pain begin?
- Is the pain there all of the time or does it come and go?
- What, if anything, makes the pain feel better?
- What, if anything, makes it feel worse?
- Are there certain times of the day or night when the pain feels better or worse?
- What other types of symptoms (e.g. stiffness, tingling, numbness, weakness, headaches) do you experience?
- Have you sustained an injury, either recently or at some time in the past, which could be related to the pain?
- Have you ever had an injury or surgery to your neck or back?
- Have you ever experienced unexplained episodes of neck or back pain in the past?
- Are you currently taking any kind of medication? If so, what kind?
- Have you experienced any problems with your bladder or bowels?
- Is there any history of osteoporosis in your family?

In addition, your doctor may enquire into the nature of your profession and your leisure activities to determine whether a strain or injury is likely, as well as into your general state of health and level of physical activity and exercise.

Physical examination

After having made a note of the medical history details surrounding your case, your doctor will then carry out a physical examination, most of which will centre around the areas of your body where you are experiencing pain or other symptoms, such as the neck, back, arms and legs. Some of the things that he or she might check for include:

- areas of pain or tenderness;
- whether there is any restriction in the movement of your spine or neck and whether there is any pain when you bend, twist or move;
- any signs of weakness in your muscles. this will typically be tested by asking you to push or lift your arm, hand or leg while the doctor applies some slight resistance;
- reflex responses in the areas below the kneecap and under the achilles tendon at the back of the ankle;
- your responses to certain sensations in specific areas, usually in the hands or feet;
- co-ordination and motor skills. you might, for example, be asked to do a toe or heel walk.

Your doctor may also carry out certain other tests which are designed to pick up signs of conditions which are directly related to the back or neck, as well as those which might stem from another source. These could include taking your temperature to check for fever, checking your pulse rate, checking your weight or testing for tenderness in certain other areas of your body.

Once the examination is complete, what happens next will depend on the doctor's findings. In some cases, the patient history and physical examination will be enough for the physician to make a confident diagnosis, in which case the next stage will be to decide upon and agree appropriate treatment. Most doctors will not automatically call for X-rays or scans to be carried out unless there are certain indicators present to suggest that these might be useful, as often these types of test do not show up anything unusual anyway. In cases where it may be beneficial, however, one of a number of different types of diagnostic test may be recommended.

Diagnostic tests

Because most cases of neck and back pain tend to clear up of their own accord within four to six weeks, generally special diagnostic tests would only be carried out after this time or in cases where the patient's history and medical examination suggest that the cause of the symptoms may be something more serious. This might be the case, for example, if the patient:

- has experienced sudden neck or back pain after a fall or other kind of accident and it is necessary to rule out a fracture;
- is experiencing back pain during the night and the doctor wishes to rule out a tumour;
- has signs of fever or is experiencing night sweats which could point to a spinal infection;
- is experiencing neck or back pain in conjunction with the loss of bladder or bowel control and/or numbness in the genital area which might indicate severe pressure on the spinal cord or nerve roots or cauda equina syndrome;
- has progressive weakness of the legs;
- either has cancer, or has had it in the past and there may be a possibility that it has spread to the spinal area.

Because children are less likely to suffer from generalised neck or back pain than adults, doctors are also usually more inclined to call for further diagnostic tests in cases involving young children and adolescents. For children and adults alike, however, depending upon the suspected cause of the neck or back pain, the tests might include one or more of the following.

X-ray

X-rays are a type of radiation, which is basically any type of energy which can travel through space as either a wave or a particle. They are similar to light but have a much higher frequency which allows them to pass through the human body, making them ideal for carrying out diagnostic tests to examine inside the body. They are very effective in terms of detecting problems with bones, such as fractures or bone infections, as well as tumours.

Having an X-ray taken is a painless process which provides a picture of the area under investigation. The patient is either asked to stand or lie very still and hold certain positions while the photographs of the spine are taken and the images are then used by the doctor to detect the nature and extent of any problems found.

Magnetic resonance imaging (MRI) scan

Magnetic resonance imaging (MRI) is also used to see internal structures of the body, such as bone, discs, ligaments and nerves, but unlike an X-ray it does not use radiation. Instead, it uses magnetic and radio waves to create images on a computer screen and is especially useful in detecting problems and changes relating to soft tissues. It can also be used to confirm lack of hydration in a disc, stenosis, a herniated disc or problems with the facet joints, as well as other problems in the back which do not necessarily originate in the spine itself.

An MRI scan normally takes between half an hour and an hour to perform and involves the patient lying on a table which slides into a machine which looks like a large, round tunnel, although newer models are not enclosed. The scanner in the machine captures many images and these are monitored by a technician and recorded for the doctor to examine and make a diagnosis.

Computed tomography (CT) scan

A computed tomography (CT) scan, which is also known as a computed axial tomography (CAT) scan, is similar to both the X-ray and the MRI scan in that it can show detailed 'slice by slice' computer images of both bones and soft tissues, but because the images are not as clear as those from X-rays or MRI scans, a CT scan is often carried out in conjunction with a myelogram. It can be useful in diagnosing problems such as the compression of a spinal nerve, spinal stenosis, disc problems and wear and tear of the bones.

As with an MRI scan, a patient who undergoes a CT scan is asked to lie on a table which slides into a scanner. As the scanner rotates, it captures images which are monitored and recorded. Again, the process takes between half an hour and an hour.

Bone scan

Bone scans are particularly useful for diagnosing precisely where in the spine a problem exists. A radioactive chemical known as a 'tracer' is injected into the bloodstream and then attaches itself to areas of bone which are undergoing changes. As the tracer accumulates in the problem area, it shows up as a dark spot which is easily detectable using a special camera. Once the right area has been identified, further tests can then be carried out which focus more specifically on this location in the body.

Bone scans are particularly useful in cases where a spinal tumour, infection or compression fracture is suspected. They are also very effective at assessing bone density and so are ideal for diagnosing osteoporosis.

Myelography
Myelography is an older technique which has largely been replaced by MRI and CT scans because of its invasive nature and increased risk of complications. It can be useful in the diagnosis of spinal nerve compression, but in cases where it is still used nowadays it is often followed by a CT scan.

In order for a myelogram to be carried out, a special X-ray dye is first injected into the patient's spinal canal using a small needle. As the patient lies on a tilting table, X-rays are taken which show the flow of the dye through the spinal region. As the dye outlines the spinal cord and the nerve roots, it becomes possible for the doctor to identify problems with the bone or discs, as well as signs of injury or tumours.

Electromyography
Electromyography (EMG) is especially useful where the function of the nerves needs to be tested and it is often used in cases where back pain radiates down the leg and is continuous or where there appears to be weakness in the muscles. The test is carried out by inserting tiny electrodes into the muscles of the lower extremity and then studying the response time of the muscle. In this way, the doctor can tell whether a nerve is being pinched or irritated.

Discography
Although discography is an invasive procedure, it can be a useful pre-operative tool to confirm that a particular disc is damaged and the source of the pain. The test involves the injection of a dye into the

centre of the damaged disc and then a spinal X-ray. As the dye makes the disc much clearer, a discogram is a much better test than either an ordinary X-ray or a myelogram.

The whole procedure normally takes around 40 minutes to perform and the patient is given medication to help them relax, followed by a local anaesthetic.

Somatosensory evoked potential (SSEP)

Somatosensory evoked potential, or SSEP as it is more commonly known, shows whether the spinal cord or nerves are being compressed, to what extent they might be damaged and whether there is, for example, a herniated or bulging disc or a bone spur causing pressure. It works by testing how well electrical signals such as touch, temperature and pain travel from the body to the brain and is performed by placing an electrode over the skin or inserting a needle into the nerve or sensory centre of the brain to measure the time taken for an electrical signal to travel through the nerve pathway. If it takes longer than expected, then it suggests that the nerve is being pinched.

Unlike some of the other tests that I have described, SSEP does not actually show the doctor what is causing the problem, but simply indicates that a problem exists. It does, however, show the doctor where to look further, which may not be within the spine itself.

Facet joint block

The principle of a facet joint block is extremely simple. Basically, in cases where the facet joint is suspected to be the problem, the doctor injects a local anaesthetic such as lidocaine or procaine hydrochloride (the latter of which is better known by the trade name Novocaine) into the joint and if the pain is alleviated it can be assumed that the diagnosis was correct. If it does not, then further tests may need to be carried out to identify the true source.

Laboratory tests

In addition to one or more of the diagnostic tests described, doctors will in some cases also carry out certain laboratory tests such as blood tests. Although these cannot detect problems caused by fractures or general wear and tear on the spine, they can help in the diagnosis of such things as infections, arthritis and cancer. In conditions such as ankylosing spondylitis where there is believed to be a genetic link, blood tests can also identify whether the suspect gene is present or not, and doctors can then follow up with X-rays, MRIs and CT scans to confirm their diagnosis.

Lumbar puncture

Another procedure which may be carried out in certain circumstances is a lumbar puncture, commonly known as a spinal tap. A lumbar puncture is actually a procedure which involves inserting a small hollow needle into the spinal canal in the lower back to extract a sample of cerebrospinal fluid and measure the pressure of the flow, followed by a laboratory test to examine the sample.

Cerebrospinal fluid flows through a channel between the layers of tissue which cover the brain and the spinal cord, helping to cushion them against sudden jarring and minor injury. The fluid is normally clear and colourless in appearance and contains few red or white blood cells. If analysis of the sample indicates any variation to this norm, therefore, it can give doctors a good indication that a certain disorder is present in the body. Although it is not a helpful test if your doctor suspects a condition such as a herniated disc, arthritis of the spine or spinal stenosis, it can be extremely useful in diagnosing infections, tumours and haemorrhaging around the brain or the spinal cord, for example:

- A higher than normal concentration of white blood cells suggests either an infection or inflammation of the brain and spinal cord.
- Cloudy fluid which has a very high concentration of white blood cells suggests the presence of meningitis (the infection and inflammation of the tissues which cover the brain and spinal cord) or sometimes encephalitis (the infection and inflammation of the brain).
- Low sugar levels might indicate either meningitis or cancer.
- High levels of protein may be the result of a brain injury or an injury to the spinal cord or a spinal nerve root.
- Blood in the fluid might suggest a brain haemorrhage.
- Abnormal antibodies point to an infection of multiple sclerosis.

In addition, elevated pressure of the fluid could result from a number of disorders, including brain tumours and meningitis.

Part Two

Living with Neck and Back Pain

5

The Impact of Neck and Back Pain

Talking about the causes and symptoms of neck and back pain can, in some ways, make it sound somewhat matter-of-fact. In reality, however, living with pain, and especially chronic pain, can have devastating effects on the quality of people's lives, not just in a physical sense, but also in terms of their emotional and psychological well-being.

When we read the accounts written by people who suffer from severe and chronic pain, it is probably just human nature to think that they are exaggerated and that these individuals are merely sympathy seekers or those who are inclined to feel sorry for themselves. Researchers and doctors around the world, however, will confirm that this most certainly is not the case, and one recent study even showed that the quality of life of people who suffer from chronic pain is lower than that of those with terminal illnesses. While this might be difficult to imagine, when you consider the difference in terms of, amongst other things, how seriously the condition is treated, the speed at which diagnosis and treatment are carried out, the certainty of the diagnosis and the levels of support which are offered by the medical profession and the loved ones of the patient, it is not actually very surprising.

Pain, as I said right at the start of this book, is something which is entirely personal and is experienced differently by every living being. It is not just a physical sensation either, but one which also involves the emotions. Even acute pain, such as might be experienced with an infection in a tooth, can drive a grown adult to utter despair in the short time that it takes to seek treatment. Chronic pain, of which spinal pain accounts for around 90%, however, can continue for months, years or even a whole lifetime. It is relentless, totally overwhelming and, in many cases, with the sufferer 24 hours a day, 365 days a year.

The issue of chronic pain and its effects on the quality of sufferers' lives is such a serious one that it has been the subject of much research over the years. In fact, there are even widely-accepted tools which are used to measure the impact of back and other types of chronic pain on life quality. One of the most commonly used in terms of back pain in particular, is the Sickness Impact Profile-Roland Scale, or SIP-Roland Scale for short, which is a modification of the Sickness Impact Profile which was already in existence and being used to rate the impact of various illnesses on quality of life. Using the responses to 24 statements which begin with 'Because of my back … ', it assesses the degree to which sufferers' lives are affected by their condition. If the respondent, for example, agrees with the statement, 'Because of my back, I go upstairs more slowly than usual', he or she would indicate this with a tick, and the greater the number of ticks, the higher the impact on their life quality. Far from being used merely to make an assessment, however, this and other such scales have been used to identify whether new pain medications or treatments being tested in clinical trials are able to improve the quality of life of sufferers by reducing their levels of back pain.

The ways in which neck and back pain can impact on the quality of life of the sufferer are numerous, and in fact it is hard to think of an area of life which remains unaffected. Alongside trying to deal with what can be immense amounts of pain and sometimes other quite disturbing symptoms, restrictions to mobility which make even normal daily activities difficult or even impossible and financial hardship caused by time lost at work or having to give up work, there are also the problems which frequently develop in relationships with partners, family members, friends and colleagues to deal with. What starts off as a purely physical complaint can very quickly become one which takes over every aspect of life and can frequently lead to problems with the overuse of pain medications, depression, anxiety and panic attacks.

In fact, this is another very important role that the tools aimed at assessing quality of life play in relation to chronic neck and back pain, because they help to identify those individuals who are at greatest risk of developing associated health problems. Those who report a very low quality of life as a result of restricted mobility, work or money-related problems and so on, are much more likely to experience an overall decline in health and well-being.

Of course, because the lives of sufferers are inherently unique, so too are the problems that they face in coming to terms and dealing with chronic pain conditions. Although many of the ways in which their lives are impacted are often very similar, children, adolescents and the elderly, for example, will typically have some quite different sets of concerns than those who are middle-aged. In the remainder of this chapter, therefore, I will take a look at some of the physical, mental and emotional issues that the majority of people who suffer from chronic neck and back pain find themselves faced with, as well as considering the younger and older age groups separately.

Fear

Pain is the body's way of telling us that all is not well. In some cases, such as when we stub a toe for example, we know why the pain has occurred and also that there is usually no serious damage. Rather than feeling fear, we are more likely to react with annoyance. With neck and back pain, however, not only may we have no idea what is causing the sensation, but even if we do, most of us are very well aware that it could lead to serious consequences and clearly this can make us feel very much afraid.

Even when we go to visit our GPs, the fact that they often do not carry out any kind of diagnostic test to definitively identify the root cause can leave us feeling terrified at the prospect that they have missed something much more serious. Even if further tests are carried out, in the UK at least, the patient may have to wait months to see a specialist, during which time they become increasingly worried, and even then the tests do not always provide a conclusive explanation. As the pain continues unabated, it becomes very easy for the sufferer to convince him or herself that the cause must be something dire.

Often though, the intensity of neck and back pain can be very misleading and, if it feels severe, it can be hard to accept that the cause is something relatively minor which does not require more drastic treatment. In reality, however, the pain experienced by one person with a herniated disc might be considerably greater than that felt by another individual suffering from a spinal infection, despite that in most cases the latter is far more serious.

Another reason why fear is typically such a huge issue for people who experience severe acute or chronic neck or back pain is connected with their uncertainty about the future. As the effects of their condition become increasingly obvious, they start to worry about how it will affect their children and partners, their work and their financial situations. Often they live with the daily fear that things will get progressively worse and that their lives will become totally unmanageable or, at the very least, changed beyond all recognition.

Pain and limited mobility

For some of those who experience neck or back pain, the symptoms may be mild and have little impact on the sufferer's ability to continue with normal daily activities. For others, however, the pain and/or restrictions to mobility can make for a thoroughly miserable existence if effective treatment is not sought. Even the simplest things like sitting comfortably or rising from a chair, reaching up to a shelf or bending to tie a shoe lace, which most of us take for granted, can cause immense pain even if they do not prove totally impossible. Walking even the shortest of distances can involve so much effort that it is not unusual for those with severe symptoms to confine themselves to their homes rather than face the agony ahead.

Even with fairly low-level but consistent pain, any enjoyment of life can be seriously marred, but in more severe cases, sufferers are often tempted to avoid completely what were once pleasurable activities. The struggle of getting into and out of a car or sit comfortably in a cinema or restaurant, or the upheaval involved in preparing for and going on holiday simply do not feel worth the incredible effort that these things involve. What typically happens, though, is that the individual begins to live an increasingly sedentary lifestyle and the pain and restricted movement become worse. Not only this, but when levels of activity are reduced, weight can also become an issue which adds to the problem.

Of course, one of the things that happens when a person's activities become so restricted is that they tend to become more and more dependent on others, and this is an issue that I will come back to shortly in relation to the elderly. Things that they were once able to do for themselves now require the help of others or are abandoned altogether. The effect of this, however, is that self-esteem and self-confidence start to become eroded and the individual's mental and emotional states are affected.

Pain and limited mobility caused by conditions of the neck or back do not just impact on an individual's home and family life of course, but they can also impose severe restrictions in the workplace, with almost any kind of occupation having the potential to be affected. For some, a job which involves standing might become either difficult or impossible, whereas for others, such as drivers, office workers and a whole host of others, sitting might be the problem. Manual work which involves lifting, carrying or bending might become totally out of the question depending on the disorder. While employers do have a legal obligation to make reasonable provisions to accommodate employees who become sick or are injured, there may be certain occasions where these are not sufficient to allow the individual to continue working. Once again, the prospect of having to give up work and the consequential loss of income typically do little to promote mental or emotional well-being.

Depression and anxiety

It is estimated that as many as half of those people who suffer from chronic pain conditions also suffer from depression and around 25% from both depression and anxiety. As anyone will know who has suffered from depression or anxiety, these are serious enough problems in their own right, but for chronic pain sufferers they also have the effect of increasing pain symptoms. Those who suffer from all three not only experience a poorer overall quality of life, but also miss more than twice as many days from work.

Although many people tend to think of depression as simply feeling a bit down, in fact this does not even begin to describe the sense of utter despair and hopelessness which is experienced, not to mention the whole range of other symptoms which typically go along with these feelings. To someone who is depressed, everything feels pointless and not only do they lose any sense of pleasure in the things that they used to enjoy, but there is not even any interest in normal activities and everyday life. Constant fatigue, difficulties in sleeping, loss of appetite or comfort eating, loss of libido, an inability to concentrate, irritability and restlessness are all common symptoms of the condition, and depression also causes intense feelings of guilt and inadequacy, as well as a total loss of self-confidence which frequently leads to the sufferer completely withdrawing from other people.

Although it is not known precisely what causes depression, it is often triggered by stressful life events, of which illness is one. In those who suffer with chronic pain conditions which affect and set so many limitations on various areas of their lives and to which there is no end in sight, it can be extremely easy to slide into depression and, having experienced one episode, there is even greater likelihood of suffering repeated bouts in the future.

Depression and anxiety quite often go hand in hand, but they are not the same thing at all. Anxiety is characterised by intense, constant and uncontrollable feelings of worry or fear, not just about a single event or situation, but about a whole range of different issues and often about non-specific events. Typically, someone who suffers from anxiety will not be able to tell you the last time that they felt relaxed.

Of course, everyone feels anxious at certain times in their lives, and in fact this is not only perfectly normal but it also helps to keep us safe by triggering the 'fight or flight' response. With generalised anxiety disorder, however, the feelings are often experienced all day, every day and they can significantly affect the way that the sufferer behaves. An inability to concentrate and sleeplessness are two very common symptoms of the condition, and in many cases sufferers also experience panic attacks. These brief or sudden attacks of intense terror can cause shaking, dizziness, nausea, confusion and difficulty in breathing and those who experience them will frequently go to great lengths to avoid situations which might trigger them, including by isolating themselves at home.

Not only do depression and anxiety each have their own set of physical symptoms, but the constant tensing of the muscles and

rigid postures which typically accompany the conditions also exacerbate existing pain symptoms, as well as create new ones. In Chapter 6,
I will come back to the issue of stress and its role in terms of contributing to pain, as well as looking at effective methods for dealing with
it. Because acceptance of a chronic pain condition is so crucial to
being able to live with it, this is also an issue which will be covered
in the following chapter.

Because depression and anxiety are so common in sufferers of
chronic pain, it is vital that doctors take these conditions into
account when carrying out their assessment of the patient and in
their treatment programmes. Treating the pain and other physical
symptoms in isolation can only have a limited effect if there are also
emotional or psychological issues present, and so taking a holistic
approach and treating the whole person, rather than just the
condition which is causing the neck or back pain, is essential.

Family and social relationships

As well as having sometimes devastating effects on the lives of sufferers
in a personal sense, chronic pain conditions almost inevitably impact
on the interactions and relationships that the individual has with those
around them, including partners, family members, friends and colleagues. This shows itself in a whole host of different ways and happens
for a variety of different reasons.

Pain, as I have said, is an entirely subjective thing, and of course
none of us are able to feel or fully appreciate the effects of pain on
another person. Where an individual has a huge gash in a part of their
body, however, we can at least guess that it is painful and to what
extent. Where they are suffering from a serious and potentially life-
threatening illness such as cancer, again we know from what we
have read and seen that the person must be in immense amounts of
pain. With chronic neck or back conditions though, not only are they
considered by many to be less serious in nature, but unless they are of a
type which causes a physical deformity, these disorders are 'invisible'
ones and this in itself can cause huge problems for sufferers. While
their bodies might be wracked with pain, there are no outward
signs to let other people know the extent of their suffering and this
can often mean that their condition is not taken seriously. Loved ones,

bosses and colleagues might become frustrated and impatient or even accuse the sufferer of exaggerating symptoms in order to avoid doing things that they do not want to do, simply because they do not understand what the individual is going through.

What makes this situation worse, of course, is the fact that doctors are sometimes unable to identify the precise cause of the pain. Even after having carried out a series of diagnostic tests, they may still not uncover any signs of trauma or injury, degenerative disease, infection, tumour or anything else. Again, this makes some cases of neck and back pain quite different from other illnesses or diseases which show up through tests, and not only can it lead to others failing to take the pain and other symptoms seriously or to belittle their effects, but it can also make the sufferer him or herself begin to feel like a fraud. Clearly, the potential for tensions to arise around these very fundamental perceptions is enormous.

In some more serious cases of neck and back pain where mobility becomes severely restricted, the sufferer may have great difficulty in carrying out normal daily activities and might have to rely on others to help with or take over certain tasks. This, of course, puts an added burden on to partners, family members, friends and colleagues who often already lead busy lives, and it can leave them feeling tired, irritable and sometimes resentful that the sufferer is not pulling his or her own weight. The loss of independence, however, is typically extremely frustrating for sufferers and often robs them of their self-esteem and self-confidence, not to mention making them feel guilty. In some cases, the guilt can even lead them to push their own limits to such an extent that they aggravate symptoms and make matters worse.

Pain, and especially that which is long-term and constant, almost inevitably takes its toll in terms of the sufferer's emotions, making them irritable and even downright angry. Although it might not be too difficult to hide these feelings from strangers or acquaintances, it is not nearly so easy to conceal them in front of friends and loved ones. When every interaction begins to feel as though it is filled with snappy comments or even sarcasm, then clearly relationships can begin to suffer. Often though, what appears to be whingeing or complaining is not aimed directly at the other person, but is simply a reflection of the sufferer's underlying frustrations, fears and worries. Effective communication, therefore, becomes all the more vital if misunderstandings are not to arise and if relationships are not to be seriously damaged.

Another example of where communication is so important is in relation to asking for help. What often happens in close or long-standing relationships is that people develop at least some ability to read one another's minds and intuit their needs. When situations change, however, not only do needs change along with them, but the individual develops a whole new set of signs and signals which their loved ones then cannot interpret. When someone who may have been perfectly fit, healthy and active develops a chronic pain condition, there is every chance that their level of capability will decrease. The only person who really knows to what extent, however, is the sufferer, and so it is up to him or her to ask for help when they need it if misunderstandings and bitterness are to be avoided.

Alongside the other effects on sufferers' normal daily activities, neck and back pain can also have an impact on their social lives and their interactions with friends. Constant refusals of invitations can either offend or lead to friends simply giving up and keeping their distance, and so it is important to keep things as normal as possible, but also to talk about your condition so that they understand that your rejection is not a personal one. When you do raise the subject, however, try not to monopolise the conversation and talk about nothing else and avoid complaining. Your friends are an extremely important source of love and support, so remember that they too have lives and issues which deserve your attention.

Where depression arises as the result of dealing with chronic pain, this can often lead to additional challenges for families and friends. Depression is a much misunderstood illness anyway, whatever its cause, and frequently the response of others is to tell the depressed person to 'pull themselves together'. When the individual fails to do so, because of course it is not within their capability, loved ones can often become frustrated and angry, not to mention feeling extremely distressed and helpless as they are forced to watch the person that they know and care about disappear before their eyes.

People attempt to deal with other people's depression in a variety of ways. Some try to cajole the depressed person out of their low mood and some lose patience and distance themselves. Often, they experience feelings of guilt and believe themselves to be responsible for the other's condition, which in turn leads them to tread on eggshells when they are around their loved one. None of these things, however, help anyone and if depression is an issue then professional help needs to be sought through a qualified therapist or counsellor.

The effect of chronic pain on family relationships is something which should never be underestimated, for the sake of the family and for the sake of the person who is suffering. Studies have shown that those patients who live in family environments where control, conflict and dependence are issues and levels of support or commitment low, as well as those which are poorly organised, respond less well to treatment. In addition, those whose emotional and psychological states incline them towards negative thinking or a lack of effort to control pain through cognitive and behavioural strategies are also at higher risk of suffering a reduced quality of life, indicating once again the importance of taking a holistic approach towards treatment.

Intimate relationships

As well as having to contend with a range of physical, emotional and psychological difficulties, those who suffer from chronic pain can sometimes find that their intimate relationships suffer too. Pain, discomfort and fatigue can all make any kind of sexual activity seem very unappealing and, in addition, either the neck or back condition itself or the medications used to control the symptoms can play havoc with the libido.

Although a couple's sex life might not appear to be one of the most obvious issues in relation to chronic neck and back pain, it is nevertheless a very real and important one. If left unaddressed, it can have an enormous impact on their emotional bond, as well as leading to the erosion of trust. Open and honest communication is essential in order for feelings to be aired and fears to be allayed and this in itself will help to maintain a close bond of intimacy. Talking to your doctor too, can be very helpful, as he or she will be able to explain any possible effects of your condition on your libido and adjust medications which are having an adverse effect.

From a physical perspective, couples may find that sexual positions which were once comfortable no longer are. Rather than seeing this as a restriction, it helps to view it as an opportunity to experiment. Positions which allow the sufferer to lean forwards, backwards or remain upright, for example, may cause less pain or discomfort according to the condition. Also, try to take advantage of the times of day when the pain is less severe or when you feel less tired.

Relationships with children

Children, and particularly younger children, can sometimes respond to illness in ways which parents do not expect. They might, for example, become very withdrawn or want to have little to do with the one who is sick, or they may resort to bad behaviour which is essentially aimed at attention-seeking.

Often when children withdraw in these kinds of situations it is fear or guilt which causes them to do so. If they fear that the illness is life-threatening, they may want to distance themselves to avoid being hurt or 'rejected' by the expected loss of the parent. Quite commonly, and possibly because younger children believe themselves to be the centre of the universe, they will even consider themselves responsible for the illness and their feelings of guilt and shame cause them to withdraw.

Attention-seeking behaviour, meanwhile, tends to arise simply because the affected parent no longer interacts with the child in the same ways as previously. Pain or disability might, for example, interfere with the ability to take part in rough and tumble games, perhaps walking to the park becomes too difficult or it might become impossible to pick up and carry a child any more and so he or she misses the close physical contact.

Taking the middle ground in terms of what children are told and trying to maintain a sense of normality are often the two most effective approaches. Too much information can frighten them, but leaving them to draw their own conclusions based on what they see and hear can, in some cases, be even more so. Often, the best approach is to talk to them in simple and reassuring language about what is happening and why Mummy or Daddy cannot perhaps do the things that they used to do, with careful attention being paid to letting the child know that he or she is in no way responsible.

Where physical activities become restricted, after explaining the problem to the child in a way that he or she can understand, try to think of alternative things that you can do together so that you can still share quality time, and of course do not let up on the hugs and cuddles.

Working Life

In the UK, back pain is one of the main reasons for workers taking time off and, according to the Health and Safety Executive (HSE), in the year 2003/04, 1% of the country's population was on sick leave because of a back problem on any one day and a total of almost 5 million working days were lost during the 12 month period. The Department for Work and Pensions (DWP), meanwhile, reports that back pain is the number two cause of long-term sickness.

Clearly, what these statistics show is not just that businesses experience an enormous impact as a result of neck and back pain, but huge numbers of individual sufferers and their families do too. Not only might there be financial repercussions due to time lost from work, but relationships with colleagues and employers may be affected, developmental opportunities lost when workers are unable to attend training events or take part in on-the-job learning, and both short and longer-term career prospects damaged. In more severe cases, some individuals may even have to give up work altogether, which can clearly have negative impacts on a whole range of areas of their lives.

As I mentioned earlier, one of the biggest problems with conditions of the neck or back which cause either acute or chronic pain is that they are invisible to others. In the workplace, the absence of any visible symptoms can unfortunately lead to colleagues and bosses questioning whether the condition really exists and suspecting that the sufferer might simply be 'swinging the lead' when they take time off work. If colleagues feel this way and are left to pick up additional tasks and responsibilities as a result of the absence, it can cause feelings of resentment. If bosses suspect this to be the case, clearly it can have huge repercussions in terms of the individual's professional reputation. This, of course, makes it all the more important that when an absence is necessary, the worker ensures that all the relevant company rules and regulations in terms of sickness reporting and providing doctor's notes are followed to the letter.

Put in black and white terms such as this, it might at first seem that the prospects for anyone who is both willing and able to continue working (which accounts for the majority of neck and back pain sufferers) are somewhat dire. There are, however, a couple of very important things to remember. First of all, as you can see from the HSE and DWP statistics, huge numbers of organisations employ workers who are affected by these conditions and, even if they were legally permitted to simply fire them (which they are not), it would not solve the problem. It costs companies between 30 and 50% of an entry-level employee's annual salary to replace them, 150% of that earned by a professional and between 300 and 500% of an executive level employee's yearly earnings. From a financial point of view alone, it is in a business' own interests to offer whatever support they can to ensure that the individual is able to work effectively and productively, and this is certainly the approach that the HSE promotes to employers. Secondly, as I have already intimated, businesses have a legal obligation to make reasonable accommodation for their workers and so are obliged, for example, to provide furniture or equipment which will help to lessen pain and discomfort and enable employees to continue in their roles.

In many instances, adaptations to the work environment can be made both simply and inexpensively by employers and where the company has its own Health and Safety representative, the first step would be to ask for a workstation evaluation to be carried out to assess current arrangements and any necessary changes. For others, however, even getting to and from work may cause problems, in which case it may be worthwhile discussing flexible work patterns and the possibility of working from home for part or all of the time. More and more employers are turning to these kinds of arrangements nowadays anyway, because of course today's technology does away with the need to maintain expensive office accommodation. If the nature of your job permits it, therefore, and you think it might be beneficial, do not feel afraid to raise the issue, although it is worth bearing in mind that staying as active as possible is generally better with most of these types of conditions, as well as the fact that going out to work provides an important social aspect which will be lost with a work from home arrangement.

Some types of occupation, of course, do not lend themselves at all to either flexible work patterns or workplace adaptations which would constitute 'reasonable accommodation', in which case it may become necessary to consider a change of duties within the existing organisation or a complete change of job and employer. Do remember, however, that if you change jobs, recruiters are not permitted to ask directly at an interview whether you suffer from any mental or physical disabilities, although they can enquire as to whether there is anything to stop you from fulfilling the role given reasonable accommodation if required. In addition, they are only permitted to access your medical records with your express consent.

The decision to give up work altogether is obviously a huge one which should not be taken lightly. Not only are there the financial implications to consider, but also the loss of the social aspect of work and the potential for isolation. In addition, it is not uncommon, even in those who retire naturally without any signs of ill-health, for diminished self-worth and the lack of a routine to lead to depression. Where there is no other choice or where finances do allow and it is the preferred option, therefore, it is important to ensure that mind and body are kept active and that a good support network of family and friends is maintained.

Chronic pain and children/adolescents

Although far less research has gone into the effects of neck and back pain in children and adolescents than in adults, clearly it does have effects in terms of schooling, family activities and socialisation. In addition, however, because some of the conditions which cause neck and back pain and affect mainly this age group are ones which either involve an obvious deformity or require the wearing of back braces or casts, issues of self-confidence and self-image are also more likely to arise.

In just the same way that adults sometimes need to take time off work because of severe levels of pain, so too might children lose time from school. If this happens regularly or the absence is long-term, then clearly it can have a long-lasting impact on their education, as well as on their future career prospects. Although it is essential to follow your doctor's advice and have the child refrain from all or some activity where this is recommended, in most cases neck and back problems respond better if the patient stays active and on the move. Whilst it might be tempting, therefore, to keep a child home from school when he or she complains of pain or tiredness due to sleep disturbances, usually it is better to insist that they attend. If absence from school does become necessary on the doctor's recommendation, then it is wise to contact the child's teacher to make arrangements for teaching material to be supplied for the child to do at home so that he or she does not fall behind.

Of course, where attendance at school is concerned, there are certain practical considerations which do need to be taken into account. Not only do parents themselves need to understand the medications that their children are taking, including dosages and any potential side effects, but so too do the staff at the school. If there are any recommendations for restrictions to the child's activities, then these also need to be passed on to the teaching establishment and parents should also make the school aware of any special requirements that the child might have in terms of furniture or equipment.

For children who suffer from chronic pain and restrictions to mobility, growing up in a household with brothers and sisters can be a frustrating and isolating experience. Siblings may not have much patience with their limitations, which can mean that they are excluded from family activities and left to occupy themselves. Fearful parents too can sometimes limit family activities, including outings and holidays, to avoid the sufferer experiencing pain and discomfort and this, of course, can have an impact on all of the children. Often though, it will be the child him or herself who shies away from activities with family or friends which might represent a challenge. Once again, it is essential that parents understand the true limitations of the child's condition, act on the advice of the doctor and keep things as normal as possible.

Children, of course, are renowned for their cruelty and, where they perceive others to be different in some way, their words can be especially harsh. It is a sad fact that there will always be some children who will take the odd pot-shot at those with obvious spinal deformities, problems with gait or who have to wear an appliance to correct problems with the spine. Yet generally speaking, society's attitudes are very different today than they were years ago. Most children are far more tolerant of those with disabilities, and schools often take a tough line with those who show any kind of prejudice or bullying behaviour.

In many cases, the problems that children with neck or back problems have in terms of socialisation seem to happen either because their own symptoms limit their activities, or because their levels of self-esteem and self-confidence are low. Children with chronic pain do make friends, but quite often they tend to have just one or two close and trusted friends, rather than a wider circle. Because pain symptoms, tiredness and depression can lead them to taking time away from school, the ability to make or retain social contacts can be affected.

As is often the case with adults, when children and adolescents with neck or back pain go untreated or fail to maintain a healthy lifestyle, their levels of overall fitness decrease and the potential for obesity increases. Often the activities that they take part in are inclined to be more sedentary ones and, unless active efforts are made to take part in regular exercise, their overall health and well-being can be affected. As many of their activities are not only sedentary, but also solitary, these youngsters can frequently experience depressed moods which not only affect themselves, but also their families.

Of course, getting enough quality sleep is incredibly important for children and teenagers, but one of the effects of any type of chronic pain condition is that it can often make this impossible. The resulting tiredness that they experience not only leads to irritability and depression, but also a further unwillingness to take part in social activities with friends or family and even greater isolation.

As I have said, there has been embarrassingly little research conducted into the effects of chronic pain in children and adolescents, but several limited studies do seem to indicate that girls over the age of 10 are particularly poorly affected. They seem to report more restrictions in daily living, as well as using more pain medication. As stress is known to have negative effects on levels of pain, and as adolescent girls are likely to suffer to a much greater extent from issues surrounding self-image, these findings could hardly be described as surprising.

Fear, for adults, is commonly a huge factor in relation to chronic pain conditions, and children and adolescents also are far from being immune to these feelings. Not only do they often worry about the nature and severity of their conditions but, just like adults, about the effects that it will have on the rest of their lives and their ability to live a normal life in the future. Although they may not easily vocalise their concerns, they fear, for example, that they may never be married as a result of their condition, or be able to have children or pursue a good career. With many years stretching ahead of them, their futures can, in their own minds, begin to look very bleak, causing them to feel frustration, anger and depression which can be taken out on other family members.

Dealing with children and adolescents who are experiencing physical, emotional and psychological distress as a result of chronic pain conditions can not only be extremely difficult, but totally heart-rending. The parents of these children frequently feel helpless and experience intense guilt at their inability to make things better. They often suffer higher levels of stress and anxiety and there is evidence of increased incidence of marital and financial problems in such families. Mothers in particular report restrictions to their lives, particularly their social lives, as a result of caring for their sick children, and even today it is mainly women who are expected to take time off work to attend to childcare needs when children are unable to go to school. Where family problems develop due to the stress of caring for a child in chronic pain, this can quickly lead to a Catch 22 situation where the guilt and anxiety experienced by the child leads to heightened symptoms which in turn cause greater stress and increase disharmony in the home.

Taking a multidisciplinary approach to treating children and adolescents with chronic neck and back pain is absolutely essential and allows a graded return to both physical and social activity. Pain needs to be managed using appropriate medications and therapies, but equally importantly, emotional and psychological issues need to be addressed. Psychological treatments such as cognitive behavioural therapy (CBT) are typically aimed at educating the child in terms of the link between thoughts and physical symptoms, as well as challenging the child's and the family's beliefs about pain. In addition, sufferers are trained in a variety of coping skills, including effective ways of relaxing which decrease pain levels. Although the principles of CBT are no different when applied to children as when applied to adults, the methods used do vary to take into account the child's age. Guided imagery, for example, which draws on the child's imagination and teaches techniques such as 'sending the pain away in a balloon' or 'rewiring computers' might be used for younger patients.

Even for children and adolescents (as well as adults) who experience severe levels of pain and restricted mobility or disability, a multidisciplinary approach to treatment has been shown to bring about remarkable improvements. By tackling physical, emotional and psychological issues simultaneously, a good percentage of patients improve sufficiently to return to school full-time and most experience significant improvements to the overall quality of their lives, with a consequent improvement in the lives of their families too.

Chronic pain and the elderly

Sadly, advancing age can bring with it an increased incidence of conditions which give rise to chronic pain and it is believed that a significant majority of elderly people experience pain which interferes with their normal functioning. Back pain, arthritis and osteoporosis are responsible for most of these cases and of course any one of these has the potential to have a considerable impact on the quality of sufferers' lives.

Aside from the more obvious effects on the elderly, such as the loss of independence, which many find extremely distressing, and the potential to suffer increased isolation, there are other factors which are peculiar to this age group and which can, in many cases, cause them to endure greater suffering. Three factors in particular are significant and these are related to the quality of the assessment and diagnosis of their conditions, the potential risks of certain medications which might prove helpful in younger patients and the frequent misconception that non-pharmacological treatments are ineffective in the elderly.

As we have seen, the huge range of neck and back conditions and the often similar symptoms which they present can make diagnosis very difficult for doctors. Several things, however, add to this difficulty where elderly people are concerned, including problems with communication, confusion and any co-existing sense of disorientation. The patient's detailed description of symptoms, along with a physical examination, form the basis of diagnosis, and clearly where the individual is unable to express clearly how they are being affected, this can greatly impact on the conclusions that the doctor is able to draw. In addition, diagnosis is complicated by the fact that many older people suffer from a range of different medical problems, some of which may cause similar symptoms or may aggravate the symptoms of neck or back pain.

Pain management, meanwhile, can be equally complex. Elderly people are more likely to be taking medications to treat other conditions and so great care is necessary to ensure that combinations of treatments do not produce unpleasant or even dangerous effects. As the elderly are typically more susceptible to the side effects of drugs, this too can cause problems in terms of finding the right course of treatment which will not only be effective, but also not add to their distress.

In terms of the third factor, that relating to non-pharmacological treatments, there are actually two issues. Firstly, for some reason certain doctors appear to doubt their effectiveness in older people, despite the fact that most of the therapies and alternative treatments have been around for many years and have been shown to work equally as well on various age groups. Secondly though, there is the perception of the patients themselves. Whereas younger generations tend to be quite open to alternative forms of treatment, and in many cases prefer to avoid traditional pharmaceutical drugs, the elderly can often be suspicious of anything which deviates from what they consider to be the norm.

Having said all of this, accurately diagnosing and prescribing effective treatments for elderly patients are not, and should never be considered to be insurmountable problems. In common with other age groups, older sufferers of chronic neck and back pain can also experience considerable improvements to their pain levels and their resulting quality of life in the hands of an expert practitioner.

6

Tension and Pain

Tension and pain are actually related in two quite separate ways. In the first case it is the 'guarding' of an injury or painful area of the body in an attempt to lessen the symptoms which leads to further pain, and in the second it is the stress associated with the injury or condition. In this chapter, I will look at both, as well as considering separately the issue of accepting pain.

Guarding

Guarding, or muscle guarding as it is often known, is basically the contraction of muscles to protect the body from pain or the fear of movement. It is not something which is done at a conscious level, but rather is a natural reflex. In some circumstances these muscle spasms only last for a few seconds, but when we are in constant pain, or constant fear of pain, the muscles do not just contract and then relax, but become permanently locked, setting up a self-perpetuating cycle of pain–spasm–pain.

Even without an injury, constant muscle tension will still cause pain, as you will find out if you try tensing a muscle or holding a certain position for any length of time. Over the long term, however, it can cause even greater problems as the muscle fibres become shortened and areas of tenderness develop. Some even believe that this muscle tension is what causes the tender points and trigger points which are associated with fibromyalgia and myofascial pain syndrome.

In cases where guarding occurs as the result of problems in the neck or back, what often happens is that posture and gait are affected. Poses or movements are adopted which, whilst being aimed at reducing pain or the likelihood of pain, actually force the body into unnatural or unbalanced positions. These unnatural stances then cause the structures of the body to change, causing further pain which can appear in unrelated parts of the body, as well as leading to the disproportionate development of the muscles.

Although I have spoken exclusively about muscles in terms of guarding, in fact other soft tissues such as the tendons, ligaments and fascia (the connective tissue which permeates the entire body and surrounds the muscles, blood vessels and nerves) can also be affected. The resulting inflammation, irritation and dehydration of these structures can cause debilitating pain which radiates around different parts of the body, and again this may play a significant part in the development of fibromyalgia and myofascial pain syndrome as secondary problems to neck and back pain.

Of course, once we become aware that muscles are tensed, we can consciously send a signal to tell them to relax. The problem with this in cases of long-term guarding, however, arise from the fact that it has become so habitual that, without learning how to relax properly and how to adopt healthier postures, it would be a full-time job to keep sending these messages. In addition, of course, if the muscles have become shortened or stuck, no amount of willpower alone will force them to release. There are, though, medications and other types of non-pharmacological treatments which can be used to help induce muscle relaxation.

Stress

Muscle tension in relation to stress works in just the same way as with guarding in that it is a totally natural and subconscious reaction. When we feel nervous or anxious, without being told to do so, our muscles lock. Our shoulders might go tense or our jaw locks, and if we are severely stressed whole areas of muscle can be quite severely affected.

Of course, the muscles of the body are not the only things to be affected by stress and in fact long-term stress can have some quite damaging effects. From a physical perspective alone, it can cause everything from digestive problems and skin conditions to heart and autoimmune diseases. In addition, it can lead to full-blown anxiety and depression.

As I described in the previous chapter, there are many aspects of chronic pain conditions which can cause stress, such as the fear that the condition might be life-threatening or that you might have been misdiagnosed, or family, relationship or financial problems which have arisen as a result. Whatever the cause, however, the effect is just the same. The muscles tense up and this causes existing pain levels to soar.

There are a number of ways of dealing with stress, most of which involve either avoiding it or reducing it, but of course the first step is to identify what causes you stress in the first place. A very effective way of doing this is simply by keeping a stress journal in which you note down how you feel each day and your particular triggers. Having identified them, you can then work out the best strategy to deal with them.

Avoiding stress is not always possible, but if you are conscious that certain people or situations make you tense up, then often it can be better to give these a wide berth rather than trying to tackle them head on. Of course, much will depend on how much you have invested in the relationship or activity, but if either are situations from which you are getting little in return, sometimes it is preferable to release them rather than compromise your own health. Where stress is caused by limited mobility and the piling up of tasks and responsibilities, often this can be avoided by planning in advance and introducing a much greater element of routine into your life.

In terms of reducing stress, there are any number of different therapies which can provide at least short-term relief. Massage and acupuncture, for example, are not only excellent in this respect, but they can also be an extremely effective form of pain relief. Meditation, deep-breathing exercises, music therapy, listening to relaxation tapes and even a good old-fashioned soak in a warm bath, however, can all help you to unwind and many people benefit from simply getting out of their normal environment and taking a quiet stroll, immersing themselves in a good book or a favourite pastime or watching a film or TV programme which makes them laugh.

For some people, the best way to deal with stress is simply to face it head-on. If work or financial issues arising from your condition are at the root of the problem, for instance, then schedule a meeting with your boss or bank manager to work out a solution. If there are a number of underlying reasons why you are feeling so tense, try to deal with them one at a time to avoid becoming overwhelmed. You do not have to do everything at once and every step that you do take will help to lighten your overall load.

Very often where chronic pain conditions are concerned, it is the sufferer's own expectations of themselves which give rise to their stress. They expect to be able to do all of the things that they used to be able to do, when clearly this is not realistic. Really stop and think about what needs to be done and then let go of any expectation that you will be able to do it as quickly or as well as previously. Also, ask for help when you need it rather than allowing yourself to become uptight about not being able to achieve it yourself.

If, despite having tried various methods of avoiding or reducing stress, you still find yourself struggling, there are of course anti-depressant medications which your doctor can prescribe. Although many of these can be very effective at treating panic, anxiety and depression, most do have potential side effects however. You can find out more about these types of medications in Part 3 of this book, but also be sure to discuss the matter fully with your doctor before taking them.

Accepting pain

One of the most common reasons why sufferers of chronic pain experience stress, and with it increased levels of pain, has to do with acceptance. In cases where pain and restricted mobility are significantly improved but not totally eradicated, people often find the idea of living with residual symptoms hard to accept. In living with the hope of a miracle cure, however, typically what happens is that they avoid doing things in the meantime which might actually help.

Failing to accept pain effectively means fighting against it, but as there is no way to control it, and controlling something which is uncontrollable is impossible, the only possible result can be stress and anxiety. Although it is quite natural to want to avoid painful experiences, in cases involving chronic pain, this can be counterproductive. By steering clear of activities which will involve pain, not only are further physical problems such as those affecting the muscles likely to develop, but there is also a greater likelihood of stress, anxiety and depression occurring as a result.

Within the field of pain research, there are those who firmly believe that avoiding activities which cause pain is one of the ways in which acute pain becomes chronic, and some researchers are now focusing on accepting pain and engaging in activities despite it. One study, the results of which were published in 2005, focused on 108 chronic pain patients in the UK, all of whom had suffered from pain, including lower back pain, for years and had tried a variety of different treatments without any great success. Most had used opioids and antidepressants and more than 40% of them had even had some kind of surgical treatment for their pain. In addition to gauging the level of pain acceptance in each of the patients, the researchers also gathered data on the pain itself, its impact, anxiety and depression, as well as conducting two physical tests.

The treatment programme which was used in this study was fairly intensive and took place over the course of three or four weeks depending on the patients' needs. It was designed to focus on improving function and it was a multidisciplinary programme involving doctors, nurses, physical and occupational therapists and psychologists, which was based on the acceptance of pain and acting in spite of it. The treatment itself included exercises which were designed to activate the entire body, as well as programmes to help patients develop healthy habits and find a meaningful direction in life. The psychological component, which figured strongly in the programme, included everything from relaxation techniques, meditation exercises and awareness of the body to improve functioning, to reversing habits, being more cognisant of avoidance thoughts and raising awareness of the social effects of displays of pain.

The results of the study showed that there was significant improvement across seven separate measures, namely:

- pain;
- depression;
- anxiety;
- physical disability;
- psychosocial disability;

- the number of hours of daily rest required due to pain;
- the number of pain medications.

The most dramatic improvements were experienced in areas of depression, psychosocial disability and the amount of pain-related rest required on a daily basis. In addition, however, there was also a marked improvement in patients' abilities to carry out the two physical tests which were a timed walk and a standing and sitting exercise. While the improvement was not quite as strong three months later, it was still significant compared to before the treatment and the patients also showed a higher level of acceptance and greater willingness to engage in activities despite their pain. The researchers believed that these results demonstrated strong potential for acceptance-based treatments, not least because they brought about a real improvement in the patients' lifestyles.

Whilst proper validation of this study would require a random, controlled trial using random patients to either receive the acceptance-based treatment, a different treatment or no treatment at all, the initial findings do seem to suggest that there is some basis in 'feeling the fear and doing it anyway'. It is, however, very important to point out that whilst accepting pain rather than fighting it almost certainly leads to less stress and anxiety, patients should always discuss what type of activities it is safe for them to take part in with their doctors in order to avoid further damage to the neck or back or the aggravation of existing symptoms.

7

The Prognosis

As you will have been able to see from Chapter 3, the prognoses for the various conditions which typically cause neck and back pain are highly variable, and of course will vary too from person to person, depending on a number of factors. Somebody who is overweight or suffers from severe depression or anxiety, for example, might reasonably be expected to respond less well to some types of treatment or experience higher levels of pain.

Very few sources quote statistics in terms of how long it takes for sufferers to recover from symptoms of neck or back pain, and those which do, vary so considerably that it would only be misleading to introduce them here. It is generally accepted, however, that most cases are acute (symptoms last less than three months) and many of these clear up without any kind of intervention. As we can see from the findings of the Department of Work and Pensions, however, there are still significant numbers of people who do suffer chronic pain as the result of neck or back problems and in some cases these can render patients incapable of carrying out their normal daily activities.

As we have seen from the results of the study described in the previous chapter, accepting long-term pain and remaining active in spite of it appears to bring about much more effective results and does much to improve patients' quality of life, as indeed does a positive mental attitude.

Another thing which is particularly significant, however, not only from the results of this study, but also from my own personal experience in dealing with literally thousands of chronic pain sufferers, is that a multidisciplinary approach to treatment results in a much better prognosis than any single treatment on its own. Treating pain without tackling mobility issues and posture will only ultimately end up in a recurrence of the symptoms. The same is true for treating pain in isolation, or even pain and mobility issues without addressing tension and anxiety. Both the patient's poor state of mind and the physical action of tensing the muscles will either make the other treatments less effective, or cause additional or more severe pain and mobility symptoms.

As you will see from the following chapters, the treatments which can be used to control and manage the pain associated with neck and back disorders are wide-ranging. When working alongside a qualified and experienced practitioner who is an expert in this field, a programme can be designed to incorporate appropriate treatment elements which are specific to the patient's individual needs and which will help to afford maximum pain relief and improved quality of life.

Part Three

Managing and Treating Neck and Back Pain

8

Pain Management

Living with chronic neck and back pain can have considerable adverse effects on the sufferer's life, but only in relatively few and very serious cases is it appropriate for surgery to be carried out to 'cure' the root cause of the problem and in some cases attempts to identify the cause prove to be futile. Even when medical investigations fail to turn up the underlying cause of the pain, however, clearly the patient cannot be left to suffer endlessly and this is where a whole range of conservative treatments can prove to be highly beneficial in terms of alleviating pain, restoring mobility and improving overall quality of life.

While some doctors are quite keen to prescribe painkillers and other types of pharmaceutical drugs to help reduce pain symptoms, often these alone are not sufficient to restore the sufferer's quality of life in the long term. In some cases, patients are intolerant to certain medications and suffer side effects which only add to their distress, and in addition these drugs might fail to address the problem adequately, such as in cases where compensatory behaviour has caused them to adopt postures which perpetuate the problem.

Pain management programmes are designed to tackle chronic pain conditions from a number of different angles. They are tailored to suit each individual patient depending upon the nature of their condition and their personal circumstances and they are aimed at restoring patients' quality of life to the maximum extent possible by reducing or eliminating pain and increasing mobility. Not only might they combine a number of drug- and non-drug-based and traditional and complementary treatments and therapies, but they also seek to educate the patient and address issues of lifestyle which may be directly causing problems or are responsible for aggravating them.

As you will see from the following chapter, the range of medications which might be prescribed as part of a pain management programme to help treat neck and back problems is fairly wide and not limited solely to pain-killing drugs. Some, for example, are used to deal with muscle spasms of the neck and back, soft tissue problems, inflammation or swelling, while others are designed to act on certain brain chemicals and regulate pain signals. Some medications might be administered in tablet form and others in the form of injections.

Various forms of manual therapy can prove to be an invaluable part of a well-designed pain management programme. Spinal manipulation and mobilisation and massage, for example, can not only provide considerable relief from pain symptoms, but also increase mobility. The ancient Chinese art of acupuncture too can be a highly effective method of reducing or eliminating pain, but in addition many much more modern techniques which use electrical pulses or low energy lasers can be extremely helpful in reducing inflammation, encouraging tissue repair and promoting healing, as well as in interrupting pain signals. A variety of physical supports such as special braces, cushions and pillows can also prove to be useful tools in the pain management specialist's armoury.

As we have seen, stress and guarding can also aggravate neck and back conditions and cause increased levels of pain, as well as further restrictions to mobility, and if these are not addressed as part of a wider programme of treatment, the individual is likely to continue to experience symptoms which might become progressively worse and even lead to long-term disability. Understanding stress and its effects, as well as learning relaxation techniques, is therefore an important part of managing long-term pain.

Unfortunately, the nature of neck and back pain conditions is such that the symptoms frequently cause sufferers to do the very things which prevent them from healing and from experiencing an acceptable quality of life. Pain and stiffness often cause them to restrict their normal activities to such a degree that movement becomes more and more difficult and muscles begin to waste. At the same time as their bodies become stiffer, weaker and increasingly pain-ridden due to the lack of exercise, weight gain can also become a problem which only adds to the severity of the symptoms. Exercise regimes and dietary programmes, therefore, might form part of the holistic approach to treating a neck or back problem.

In common with many chronic pain conditions, neck and back problems very often lead to emotional and psychological difficulties which can sometimes become severe and debilitating in themselves. Fear of what the future may hold, lifestyle restrictions, isolation due to limited mobility, relationship difficulties which arise from or are aggravated by the condition, not to mention the sheer misery of living in constant and sometimes severe pain, can all take their toll on mental and emotional health and ultimately lead to depression and/or anxiety. Again, these only serve to increase physical suffering if they are not treated as part of an overall programme and so a pain management specialist might also recommend some kind of psychotherapeutic treatment, such as cognitive behavioural therapy (CBT), as part of a multi-faceted treatment plan.

Specialist pain management clinics aim to teach sufferers of chronic pain how to manage their symptoms, as well as how to increase their activities and ensure a better quality of life. Rather than their recommended programmes being rigid and set in stone, they monitor carefully what is and is not working for the patient so that adjustments can be made and the most effective treatment ensured. Medications might be altered if these fail to bring about the desired results, and of course practitioners work with patients to ensure the right balance and combination of exercise and physical therapies, as well as drawing on alternative treatments and therapies as required.

Because pain management clinics treat neck and back pain using a variety of different techniques as appropriate to the individual patient, they are staffed by a range of practitioners who are all specialists in their fields. With a particular interest in their own disciplines, each remains at the cutting edge in terms of new developments in understanding and treatment. Rather than working in isolation, however, in this environment a fully trained and qualified interdisciplinary team of pain management consultants, medical practitioners, physiotherapists, psychologists, occupational therapists and nurses work hand in hand with their colleagues to ensure the most effective combinations of treatment possible.

In the remainder of this part of the book, you will find information relating to the wide variety of treatments and therapies which might be employed as part of a pain management programme, as well as some useful self-help tips which are aimed at ensuring your own improved quality of life.

9

Medications and Contraindications

Prescribed and over-the-counter medications are often the mainstay of general practitioners when treating both acute and chronic cases of neck and back pain. In some cases involving acute pain caused by, for example, a minor sprain or strain, they may be all that is required to relieve symptoms and restore the patient to an acceptable quality of life until the body has had the chance to heal naturally. In cases involving certain conditions or those in which the pain and other symptoms progress and become chronic in nature, however, often their use is much more effective when they are given a supporting role as part of a wider-ranging treatment programme, rather than being used in isolation.

Medications can provide a number of benefits in relation to cases of neck and back pain. Not only can they be used to directly or indirectly relieve pain or other symptoms, but in helping to alleviate sources of discomfort, they can also make other elements of a multidisciplinary pain management programme more possible. By reducing levels of pain, for example, the patient will be more motivated and better able to take part in exercise programmes designed to restore mobility and encourage beneficial weight loss. In this way, the individual experiences improvements from a number of different sources which together have a much more significant impact on quality of life.

Treatment for neck and back pain which relies solely on medication and goes on for a prolonged period of time can cause problems in itself. If prescribed doses are insufficient to provide acceptable levels of relief from pain or the effects lessen over time, then there is the risk that the sufferer might begin to self-medicate, either by increasing the recommended dosage, increasing the frequency of doses, supplementing prescribed medications with other over-the-counter drugs or even turning to illicit drugs or alcohol as a means of numbing their symptoms. In addition, if there is any expectation on the part of the patient that medication is the sole remedy, then he or she is highly unlikely to address issues such as education, acceptance, posture, exercise, weight loss and depression which, if tackled simultaneously, could all have the potential to provide significant relief and offer vast improvements to the quality of life.

Having said this though, as part of a holistic approach to pain management, medicinal treatments do undoubtedly have an important part to play in many instances. Understanding the role of different types of medications, as well as any possible side effects and the potential for different types of drugs to react with one another, however, is important if the best single drug treatment or combinations of treatment are to be identified.

The four main types of medication which are used to treat neck and back pain are designed to:

- relieve pain;
- reduce inflammation and swelling;
- relax the muscles;
- alter the perception of pain.

In the remainder of this chapter, you will find descriptions of oral and topical medications which are commonly prescribed to achieve these aims and how they work, as well as any contraindications or potential side effects to the drugs. In addition, I will then look at some of the types of injection which also prove to be useful in achieving some of the same ends.

Painkillers and anti-inflammatory drugs

Analgesics and non-steroidal anti-inflammatory drugs (NSAIDs) are some of the most commonly used medications for neck and back pain. In certain situations, corticosteroids may also be administered in tablet form, although these can also be delivered by means of an injection. All of these drugs work in different ways, and while analgesics act solely to relieve pain, NSAIDs and corticosteroids also act to reduce inflammation.

Analgesics

The two main types of analgesic are those containing acetaminophen, such as Tylenol, which can generally be bought over-the-counter, and opioids which are prescription-only drugs.

Acetaminophen, which is more commonly known as paracetamol, is widely used to treat mild to moderate neck or back pain, as well as a variety of other muscle aches, headaches, toothache, period pains, fevers and the general aches and pains which typically accompany colds and flu. It targets pain by inhibiting the production of pain chemicals in the body and altering the way that pain signals are processed by the brain. It is available in the form of tablets, suspensions, rapidly-dissolving or chewable tablets, effervescent tablets or granules, as well as in rectal suppository form.

Although it is a widely and easily available drug, which tends to suggest that it is also totally safe, acetaminophen can cause damage to the liver if it is taken in excessive doses or over prolonged periods of time. It is therefore essential that the directions on the packaging are followed closely or that the drug is taken as directed by your doctor. Because both the drug itself and alcohol can damage the liver, anyone with a history of alcoholism or who drinks more than three alcoholic beverages per day should inform their doctor before taking acetaminophen, as well as those who have, or have ever had, alcohol or non-alcohol-related liver disease, as it may not be safe for you to take this form of medication. Advice should also be sought by pregnant women and nursing mothers as the effects of the drug on unborn children are unknown and nursing babies may be harmed by the passing of acetaminophen into the breast milk.

One of the important things to remember about acetaminophen or paracetamol is that it is a common ingredient in many other medications such as other painkillers, cold remedies, allergy medicines and sleep medications. Always check with your doctor or pharmacist, therefore, to ensure that your overall dosage of the drug is not exceeded. Acetaminophen is also available in prescription-only form where it is combined with narcotic analgesics.

Opioids, which are a much stronger class of drugs used to treat severe and chronic pain, are only available on prescription. They work by binding themselves to the opioid receptors in the central and peripheral nervous system and the gastrointestinal tract to reduce the body's perception and reaction to pain and increase pain tolerance. The group of opioid drugs includes synthetically produced medications such as meperidine (Demerol) and tramadol (Ultram), as well as morphine and codeine which are derived from opium. Some opioids are combined with paracetamol to make them work better, so that, for example, codeine and paracetamol are combined to produce co-codamol and tramadol and paracetamol are combined to make tramacet. Even though opioids are stronger than some other forms of medication, this does not necessarily mean that they will eradicate pain altogether and still they are most effective when used as part of a multidisciplinary pain management programme.

Those patients who are prescribed opioids sometimes experience a range of side effects which usually last for several days but can go on for longer. These might include:

- dizziness;
- nausea and/or vomiting;
- drowsiness;
- dry mouth;
- weakness;
- headaches.

Longer-term use, on the other hand, can lead to:

- constipation;
- weight gain;
- itching;
- loss of libido;
- difficulty breathing at night.

High doses taken over many months or years can cause:

- low libido;
- reduced fertility;
- irregular menstruation;

- erectile dysfunction;
- reduced ability to fight infection;
- increased levels of pain.

Patients who suffer from respiratory depression, including as a result of the condition known as sleep apnoea, in which the muscles and soft tissues of the throat relax and collapse sufficiently to cause a total blockage of the airway, may not be prescribed opioids because of the additional breathing difficulties that the drugs can cause. In addition, great care needs to be taken in prescribing these drugs to pregnant women as the baby may develop breathing difficulties at birth or suffer from the symptoms of opioid withdrawal.

One of the main problems with opioids is that they tend to become less effective over time as the body develops a tolerance to them, and in some cases patients even develop a cross tolerance, so that prolonged use of one opioid results in a tolerance to all of the drugs in this group. Dependence on opioids can also occur, so that when patients stop taking the drug suddenly or reduce the dose too quickly, withdrawal symptoms are likely to be felt. It is important, therefore, that discontinuation of the drug is directed and supervised by a medical professional and that patients are careful not to run out of their medication if they are to avoid symptoms which might include:

- sweating;
- runny nose;
- stomach cramps;
- tiredness;
- diarrhoea;
- muscle aches.

Although addiction to opioids amongst chronic pain patients is thought to be rare, those who have been addicted to opioids, other drugs or alcohol and those suffering from severe depression or anxiety are believed to be at greater risk.

Non-steroidal anti-Inflammatory drugs (NSAIDs)

Non-steroidal anti-inflammatory drugs (NSAIDs) are not only highly effective at easing pain, but also at reducing inflammation, which is a common component of neck and back-related pain. They are used to treat a range of painful conditions and many of those who suffer from neck and back pain find them more useful than paracetamol or opioids. Although some NSAIDs are only available on prescription, two of the most common, aspirin and ibuprofen, are available as over-the-counter preparations.

NSAIDs work by preventing both forms of the enzyme cyclooxygenase, known as COX-1 and COX-2, from doing their job. COX-1 is what protects the lining of the stomach from digestive chemicals and acids, as well as helping to maintain the proper functioning of the kidneys, and COX-2 is a protein which is produced when the joints become inflamed or injured. At the same time as doing a highly effective job of easing pain and inflammation, therefore, they can also increase the risk of nausea, stomach upsets, stomach ulcers and bleeding inside the stomach, as well as having adverse effects on kidney function, especially if taken over prolonged periods of time. Those with existing stomach ulcers or who have a history of kidney or liver disease, heart problems, asthma or high blood pressure may not be able to take standard forms of NSAIDs at all, or these might only be prescribed in very low doses, and even those for whom these are not issues should still take such medications with food to minimise the potential for side effects.

Although still not suitable for those with a history of heart disease or pregnant women, a newer form of NSAIDs known as COX-2 inhibitors which have a less harmful effect on the stomach may be prescribed for some patients, although they are not available over the counter. These drugs, one of the most common of which is Celebrex, do not eliminate the potential gastrointestinal side effects altogether, but they do reduce them considerably and so are considered much safer. They do, however, come with their own set of potential side effects, including:

- indigestion;
- abdominal pain;
- nausea;
- headaches;
- dizziness;
- weakness;

- fatigue;
- increased risk of heart attack;
- increased risk of blood clots.

Whether your doctor is considering prescribing either traditional NSAIDs or COX-2 inhibitors for neck or back pain, always be sure to disclose any past or current problems such as:

- gastrointestinal problems;
- heart attacks;
- strokes;
- angina;
- blood clots;
- high blood pressure;
- sensitivity to aspirin or any other NSAIDs.

It is also important that you do not take a prescription or over-the-counter form of a traditional NSAID at the same time as a COX-2 inhibitor.

In cases where neck or back pain is caused by problems with the bones in the spine, another thing which is well worth discussing with your doctor is the impact of NSAIDs and COX-2 inhibitors on the ability of the bone to heal, as some studies have shown that these drugs can slow down the healing process if used for any significant amount of time.

Corticosteroids

Corticosteroids, which are often known simply as 'steroids', are not to be confused with the steroids which are sometimes taken by sportsmen and women to improve their performance or by body builders to help them pack on muscle. In fact, these drugs are sometimes prescribed by doctors to control and reduce painful inflammation and, although often administered by injection, can also be taken orally in tablet form. Pain which emanates from the nerve root and is caused, for example, by a herniated disc or spinal stenosis which is characterised by the narrowing of the spinal canal, or cases in which rheumatoid arthritis affects the spine, might respond well to this type of medication.

Corticosteroids are steroid hormones which are produced naturally in the body and play a part in the functioning of a variety of the body's systems, one of which is responsible for regulating inflammation. The synthetic corticosteroids used to treat a range of conditions which encompasses everything from brain tumours to skin conditions, are pharmaceutical drugs which act in a similar way to the naturally produced hormones, but they are very powerful drugs which can cause some serious side effects.

Probably the most widely known side effect of steroids is one which impacts on children and teenagers. In this age group, these medications can slow or even stop growth, as well as affecting the adrenal glands which naturally secrete the hormone. In addition, the administration of corticosteroids to youngsters can also lead to childhood illnesses such as measles and chickenpox being much more serious than they might otherwise have been, so doctors and parents of children with neck and back problems need to seriously consider whether the benefits of the drug truly outweigh any potential side effects which may result.

Another group of patients who can be adversely affected by corticosteroids is the older age group. High blood pressure and bone disease are two of the most significant problems which can arise from the use of these medications, but long-term use can also result in:

- hyperglycaemia (high blood sugar);
- colitis;
- erectile dysfunction;
- cataracts;
- insulin resistance;
- hypothyroidism;
- anxiety;
- depression.

In older women in particular the risk of osteoporosis is significantly greater in cases where corticosteroids are taken.

Across all age groups, a variety of less serious side effects may present themselves, but medical attention should still be sought if you experience:

- stomach or abdominal pains;
- nausea and/or vomiting;
- continually runny, dry or stuffy nose;
- continually watery eyes;
- rashes, acne or other skin problems;
- loss of the sense of smell or taste;
- swelling of the face, lips or eyelids;
- any unusual bruises or marks on the skin;
- wounds which refuse to heal;
- rapid weight gain;
- sleep problems;
- increase or decrease in appetite;
- indigestion;
- pain in the eyes or problems with vision;
- unusual tiredness or weakness;
- cramps, pain or weakness in the muscles;
- black stools;
- white patches in the mouth or throat, or white patches or sores inside the nose or in the anal area;
- pain on swallowing or eating;
- menstrual problems;
- irregular heartbeat;
- mood swings;
- confusion, excitement, restlessness or nervousness;
- disturbing thoughts or feelings;
- hallucinations.

Anyone who experiences wheezing, problems with breathing or tightness in the chest should seek urgent medical attention.

As corticosteroids can create low levels of potassium and high levels of sodium in the body, those who take them over long periods of time may need to follow special low-sodium and high-protein diets. The lowered resistance to infection which tends to occur in all age groups also means that infections are more likely to occur and, when they do, they are generally harder to treat, making it important for anyone taking this type of medication to seek medical attention promptly and to advise the attending physician that they are taking corticosteroids.

Because corticosteroids can react with other types of medication, either changing the way that the drugs work or increasing the risk of side effects, it is important that your doctor be made aware of any other medicines that you are taking, including but not limited to:

■ insulin or other medicines used to treat diabetes;
■ any medication used to treat heart conditions;
■ blood thinners such as Warfarin;
■ diuretics (water pills);
■ antacids if taken frequently;
■ oral contraceptives or any drugs containing oestrogen;
■ any medications which contain potassium or sodium;
■ Cyclosporine.

Your doctor should also be advised of any recent vaccinations that you have had; if further vaccinations are planned, these should be discussed with your physician before going ahead.

Not only can certain other types of medication affect the way that corticosteroids work or increase the chances of side effects, so making the prescription of these drugs inadvisable, but people who suffer from certain other conditions also need to ensure that their doctors are aware of their pre-existing medical problems. These include people with:

■ any type of viral, bacterial or fungal infection;
■ hypo or hyperthyroidism;
■ stomach or intestinal problems;
■ diabetes;
■ high blood pressure;
■ glaucoma or cataracts;
■ high cholesterol;
■ osteoporosis;
■ current or past tuberculosis;
■ heart disease;
■ liver disease;
■ kidney disease;
■ kidney stones;
■ conditions which cause the skin to bruise easily or become thinner;
■ systemic lupus;

- myasthenia gravis;
- emotional problems.

Those who have experienced allergic or unusual reactions to corticosteroids in the past should also discuss these with their physicians, as should pregnant women and nursing mothers. Although inhalant and nasal forms of the drugs are considered to be safer than oral or injected forms, excessive use in any form can affect a baby's growth rate after birth and whilst being breastfed.

Muscle relaxants

Muscle relaxants essentially fall into two major groups. While the group of neuromuscular-blocking drugs is used to paralyse muscles by blocking the transmission of nervous signals and is typically used during surgery and intubation, skeletal muscle relaxants such as benzodiazepines and methocarbamol work on the central nervous system and relax the muscles to a much lesser extent. In the case of conditions which cause neck and back pain, the latter are typically used to control muscle spasms or the pain and stiffness associated with strains, sprains and other types of spinal injury, increasing mobility and range of motion. Some of the benzodiazepines are also well known for treating cases of anxiety.

Some of the most commonly used skeletal muscle relaxants include carisoprodol, cyclobenzaprine, metaxalone, diazepam and methocarbamol which typically appear under the brand names of Soma, Flexeril, Skelaxin, Valium and Robaxin respectively. All of these drugs have the potential to cause sedative effects on the patient, which means that driving or operating machinery whilst under their effects or combining their use with alcohol can be extremely hazardous, and some users experience:

- drowsiness;
- lethargy;
- dizziness;
- lightheadedness;
- changes in urine colour;
- confusion;

- nervousness or restlessness;
- irritability;
- double vision or blurred vision;
- impaired movement and co-ordination;
- dry mouth;
- heartburn;
- weakness;
- trembling;
- constipation;
- headaches;
- nausea and/or vomiting;
- stomach cramps/pains;
- upset stomach.

In most cases, these symptoms are only short-lived and improve when the body begins to adjust to their presence, but anyone experiencing any of the following should seek prompt and urgent medical attention:

- breathing difficulties;
- unusually fast or slow heartbeat;
- tightness in the chest;
- fainting;
- swelling of the face, mouth, lips or tongue;
- fever;
- chills;
- sore throat;
- rashes, itching or hives;
- stinging, red or bloodshot eyes;
- yellowing of the skin or eyes;
- unusual thoughts, feelings or dreams.

In addition, certain muscle relaxants such as diazepam also carry a high risk of dependence, particularly when taken over prolonged periods of time.

A variety of medical conditions can present problems in relation to the taking of skeletal muscle relaxants and anyone who is suffering from, or has suffered in the past with any of the following should discuss their condition with their physician before taking any of these drugs:

- diabetes;
- epilepsy;
- kidney disease;
- liver disease;
- hepatitis;
- irregular heartbeat;
- heart attack;
- allergies;
- overactive thyroid;
- glaucoma;
- urinary problems;
- alcohol abuse.

As muscle relaxants can react with other types of medication, it is also vital that you make your doctor aware of any other types of drugs that you are currently using, including over-the-counter preparations. Pregnant women and breastfeeding mothers should also exercise extreme caution in relation to muscle relaxants as there is evidence to suggest that certain of these drugs may be responsible for causing anything from sleepiness and lethargy in babies to foetal abnormalities such as cleft lip and palate.

Skeletal muscle relaxants are normally only prescribed on a short-term basis and often provide such considerable relief that patients feel tempted to return to normal activities, which in some cases can actually cause further damage. It is very important, therefore, that the use of these drugs is combined with exercise and physical therapies which are designed to bring about longer-lasting improvements to the individual's condition.

Topical medications

Alongside the oral medications that we have looked at so far, there are also numerous topical medications which are available over the counter in pharmacies or on prescription to help with certain types of neck or back pain. Pain which arises from the muscles due to strains, sprains or other types of injury, or as a result of osteoarthritis, rheumatoid arthritis or some types of nerve pain, for example, might respond well to topical medications. However, pain caused by a herniated disc or narrowing of the spinal column or that which originates deep inside the body is unlikely to be much affected.

Topical medications come in a variety of different forms including creams, ointments, gels, patches and sprays and these represent a fairly efficient way to deliver analgesic, anaesthetic or anti-inflammatory drugs, including corticosteroids, to the site of the pain. Because the skin is the largest organ of the human body with blood vessels and nerve endings lying just below its surface, it can carry the medication quickly and accurately to the pain source so that relief from symptoms is normally achieved more quickly than with oral medicines. As the drug initially bypasses the digestive system, the stomach problems that some patients suffer with the likes of NSAIDs, for instance, can often be reduced if not eliminated altogether. In many cases, the amount of the drug which is required to achieve the same effect is less when it is applied topically, but relief from symptoms can last longer as the drug is released at a steadier rate.

Like oral medications, topical medications are not without their drawbacks however. Because the drug is applied to the skin and absorbed via a 'carrier', there is the potential for skin reactions or allergies to occur. In addition, because blood flow is not only different to different areas of the body, but also because it changes according to, for example, temperature, patients often need to be properly educated in terms of where, how and when it should be applied to achieve maximum benefit. Having said this though, because topical medications delivered in patch form, for instance, provide a slow release of the relevant drug, many find these much more convenient than having to swallow tablets every few hours.

Injections

Although some patients are terrified at the prospect of any kind of injection, one of their greatest benefits for those suffering from pain is the ability to deliver the required medication directly to the source of the problem. Clearly, great care is taken by medical staff when delivering injections to the spinal area, and the procedure is often performed in an X-ray department so that the specialist can position the needle accurately and safely.

Most injections which are given to alleviate neck and back pain contain corticosteroids to reduce inflammation, often combined with an anaesthetic. Depending upon the nature of the condition, they might be delivered into the soft tissues, the epidural space in the outermost part of the spinal canal or in the exact location of the nerve root. Epidural steroid injections are most commonly used to treat those who are suffering from herniated discs or spinal stenosis (narrowing of the spinal canal), and are also particularly useful for conditions such as arthritis of the facet joints and degenerative disc disease.

Nerve block injections, the type of which are done in the location of the nerve root, are often used to serve a dual purpose. As well as being very effective in the treatment of nerve pain, they are also very useful in terms of diagnosing the precise cause and location of the pain. Basically, if the injection works by alleviating inflammation around the nerve root, so reducing or eliminating pain, then the specialist can be assured that it originates from a specific nerve. If it has no effect, however, then he or she will know to continue investigations elsewhere.

Trigger point injections are another type which may be appropriate in certain circumstances. Trigger points are basically tight nodules in the muscles which produce tenderness or twitching when touched or pressurised and can cause either localised or referred pain. These painful areas of muscle can occur as the result of accidents or injuries in which muscles stretch and contract suddenly and violently or in cases where muscles become overused, such as might be the case when patients adopt compensatory postures or gaits or guarding positions to avoid experiencing pain to an injured area of the body.

The extent of the pain relief achieved through injections can vary hugely. In some cases, they may need to be repeated within a matter of 10 days to two weeks, whereas in others the effects might last for several months. A relatively new type of injection which has so far been shown to provide excellent and much longer-lasting results in patients suffering from painful muscle spasms and 'knots' is that containing Botox. Although most commonly associated with cosmetic procedures designed to hold back the ravages of time and smooth out wrinkles, the drug can also be used in a medical sense to block neuromuscular transmission and cause the selective weakening and paralysis of muscles which alleviates pain and spasms.

Botox is actually made from a toxin produced by the bacterium called Clostridium botulinum, although clearly it is purified before being used for either cosmetic or medical purposes and even then it is only used in very small quantities. Because it can have devastating effects on the nervous system in the wrong hands, it is vital that patients are only treated with the drug by licensed physicians who have experience of working with Botox and can administer it safely, in which case they can expect to achieve very significant results. Although in some cases it may take between one and three weeks for the effects of the drug to kick in, relief from pain symptoms typically lasts for two to four months, with studies showing that a significant majority of sufferers experience significant reduction in pain levels and increased range of movement.

Of course, where injections in general are concerned, the same contraindications and side effects apply to these as to their oral equivalents. In the case of corticosteroid injections, for example, when the medication is absorbed into the body following an injection, there is the same risk that the individual's ability to fight infection may be compromised or that the body's blood sugar levels might be affected. In the same way that people with diabetes or heart problems might not be considered suitable for taking corticosteroids by mouth, therefore, they may also not be suitable candidates for corticosteroid injections. In the case of Botox injections, however, after effects or side effects from the drug have been found to be rare and only minor, with those affected comparing them to flu-like symptoms. As is the case when any type of medication is being considered though, those considering Botox injections should discuss their current and past medical history with their physician before going ahead to ensure that the procedure is entirely safe and appropriate.

As well as thinking about the drug contained within the injection itself, another thing worth bearing in mind with injections is the fact that these are invasive and there are additional risks associated with introducing a needle into such a sensitive area as the spine. Although injections are carried out in a sterile environment, there is still a small risk of infection being introduced into the body, which can lead to quite severe consequences in cases where the spine itself is affected. Another fairly rare (0.1–5% occurrence) but possible complication of an epidural steroid injection is a dural puncture, where spinal fluid continues to leak from the spinal sac which fails to seal itself. The decreased pressure of the spinal fluid in the brain, which causes what can be severe headaches and nausea, is usually treated by injecting several ounces of blood taken from the arm into the epidural space. As the blood clots around the spinal sac, it effectively forms a patch to stop the leak.

Accidental injection into one of the tiny blood vessels which runs through the epidural space is another possible risk, and in cases where too much of the medication enters the bloodstream this can be serious. Although the chances of this happening are only slight, it can result in seizures, cardiac arrest or even death. Where a blood vessel is damaged in the course of the injection, this can also cause internal bleeding, which if it puts significant pressure on the nerves of the spine, can cause bladder and bowel problems to develop. Damage to the spinal nerves with the epidural needle, meanwhile, can result in permanent injury.

Although the chances of something going wrong in the course of administering spinal injections are relatively low, it is vitally important that patients only put themselves in the hands of practitioners who are fully trained, qualified and experienced in treating neck and back conditions.

Other medications

Tricyclic antidepressants

Alongside painkilling medications, non-steroidal anti-inflammatory drugs (NSAIDs) and muscle relaxants, another group of drugs which is sometimes used to treat cases of chronic pain, is that containing the tricyclic antidepressants. Although, as the name suggests, these were originally developed to treat depression, at lower doses they can sometimes prove to be highly effective for chronic pain conditions which do not respond to other types of treatment.

Quite how tricyclic antidepressants work to reduce levels of pain is not entirely understood by the medical profession, although the fact that they restore the balance of certain chemicals in the brain, such as serotonin, norepinephrine and dopamine, and contribute to more restful sleep may all improve the sufferer's ability to cope with pain. Because they induce drowsiness, it may also be the case that patients are better able to relax formerly tense muscles, which in itself can help to relieve pain. Certainly in cases involving conditions such as rheumatoid arthritis and spondylosis, however, they have shown to be particularly effective.

One of the most widely used tricyclic antidepressants is amitriptyline, although desipramine, doxepin, imipramine, amoxapine and nortriptyline, all of which are marketed under a variety of different brand names, may also be prescribed. Unlike in cases where these drugs are prescribed at higher doses and specifically to treat depression, the side effects experienced by those with chronic pain conditions who take lower doses tend to be less troublesome, although they can include:

- drowsiness;
- dizziness;
- nausea;
- dry mouth;
- dry eyes;
- sweating;
- problems passing urine;
- constipation;
- changes in weight.

Generally, these side effects ease within 7–10 days as the body adjusts to the presence of the drug, but if they do continue or become troublesome, then talk to your doctor who may be able to prescribe a different antidepressant which suits you better. Of course, in common with other medications, anyone who experiences drowsiness or dizziness should not drive or operate machinery, and alcohol should also be avoided as this is likely to increase the sensations.

More serious side effects are rarer, but if you experience any of the following then it is important to seek medical help immediately:

- increased heart rate;
- sudden numbness;
- sudden headache;
- blurred vision.

Another significant side effect reported by some who take amitriptyline in particular is a tendency towards sudden suicidal thoughts. Again, should this be the case, contact your doctor or go to your nearest hospital immediately.

Serotonin and norepinephrine reuptake inhibitors

Another type of antidepressant that you may be prescribed belongs to the group of serotonin and norepinephrine reuptake inhibitors, or SNRIs for short. These drugs work by increasing the levels of serotonin and norepinephrine by stopping them from being reabsorbed into the brain. As these chemicals are responsible for maintaining a healthy mental balance, again it may be that patients feel more relaxed and better able to deal with pain, so that the pain feels less severe. Duloxetine, which is most often seen under the brand name of Cymbalta, is one of the most commonly used SNRIs.

Whereas tricyclic antidepressants tend to aid restful sleep, one of the side effects of SNRIs is that they can cause insomnia in some people, in which case doctors may prescribe a tricyclic antidepressant as well. Drowsiness and dizziness, however, may also result from taking SNRIs, but again if you experience blurred vision or extreme nausea, then you should seek urgent medical attention. Patients who are already taking non-steroidal anti-inflammatory drugs (NSAIDs), aspirin or blood thinners such as warfarin should also be especially careful to make their doctors aware of this, as the combination of these with SNRIs can increase the risk of haemorrhage.

Selective serotonin reuptake inhibitors

Selective serotonin reuptake inhibitors (SSRIs) are some of the newest types of antidepressants on the market. In much the same way as SNRIs, these work by preventing the reabsorption of the chemical neurotransmitter serotonin into the brain so that the perception of pain is less. SSRIs, however, do not have any impact on levels of norepinephrine and so are sometimes considered to be less consistently effective.

Although some may not be familiar with the term SSRI, few will not have heard of the drug Prozac, which is one of the most commonly prescribed of this group of drugs. Zoloft, Paxil and Luvox are other brand names which you might come across too.

Again as with SNRIs, although many people who take SSRIs experience drowsiness, some find that it causes sleep disturbances and so may also be prescribed a tricyclic antidepressant to counteract this side effect. Other side effects might include nausea, dry mouth and/or weight gain, but should increased heart rate or seizures be the result of taking one of these medications, then medical help should be sought immediately.

Bone growth medications

While all of the different types of medications that we have looked at so far have been aimed, in one way or another, at reducing or eliminating the pain associated with neck and back conditions, there are other drugs which are designed to prevent or delay the effects of the underlying condition. Examples of these include a range of drugs which are used to treat osteoporosis by stimulating the cells (osteoblasts) which form new bone, slowing down the cells (osteoclasts) which break down bone, or both.

New drugs such as Actonel which claim to prevent and treat osteoporosis by increasing bone mass and preventing bone fractures are becoming increasingly popular. By working alongside a pain management specialist who is at the forefront of discovery and innovation, patients who suffer from neck and back pain can benefit from all the latest developments in relation to medications and other forms of treatment.

Case Study 1

A 61-year-old lady who was suffering from lower back pain was seen at the London Pain Clinic and upon examination she was found to be experiencing extreme tenderness of the right sacroiliac joint and some right lumbar facet joint tenderness. The patient was immediately put on the list for X-ray guided injections to help with these problems. In addition, we also discussed certain activities that the patient was involved in, including yoga, ballet and football. I advised her that even if we were able to find a pain-free window, it would be best to moderate the extent of these activities as they were likely to exacerbate the pain. During the time that she was waiting for the injections to be carried out, the lady began using Celecoxib anti-inflammatory medication which proved to offer some relief.

When the lady returned to the clinic, she was given right L3/4, L4/5 L5/S1 and right sacroiliac joint injections containing Bupivacaine 0.25% 20 ml and 80 mg of Depo-Medrone. The injections were given under X-ray guidance. Although the results of the procedure appeared to be unremarkable at first, when the patient was reviewed at the clinic two months later, the pain had completely resolved and she was discharged.

Case Study 2

I reviewed the case of a 52 year-old gentleman who had a history of neck and lower back pain and whose recent MRI scan showed a slight cervical intervertebral disc protrusion. On examination, I found that he experienced tingling in both hands, which was said to be felt on a daily basis and more in the right hand than the left. Examination of the neck revealed a reduction in flexion and marked reduction of extension and lateral rotation produced by pain. No abnormality was detected in tone and power and light touch was normal, but reflexes were reduced on both the left and the right. The patient was taking the compound analgesics co-codamol and co-dydramol, as well as the tricyclic anti-depressant nortriptyline as required.

My clinical impression was that this gentleman was suffering from cervical facet joint tenderness, which was most likely secondary to a small cervical disc protrusion and secondary myofascial pain syndrome. He also had lumbar facet joint tenderness and I noted that he had had a mini spine operation to remove fibrous tissue from the nerve root and L4.

In the first instance, the patient was given anti-inflammatory drugs in the form of Etoricoxib 90 mg as required and he was booked in for X-ray guided cervical facet joint injections. The injections were performed on the left at C3/4, C4/5 and C6/7 and on the right at C4/5 and C6/7 and a total of 20 mls of 0.5% Bupivacaine and 80 mg of Depo-Medrone were used.

When reviewed at the clinic two months later, the patient was doing extremely well. He had stopped taking all of his analgesics and found that the pain had dramatically reduced. He had also started his physiotherapy-based rehabilitation, including aerobic exercises and postural retraining. He found this treatment to be extremely helpful and, given the improvement, he was discharged from the clinic.

10

The Role of Physiotherapy

For anyone suffering from severe and/or chronic pain, the top priority will almost certainly be to eradicate, or at the very least reduce the discomfort, and in the previous chapter I outlined some of the main pharmaceutical drugs which are used to achieve this. As you will have seen, however, in almost every case both over-the-counter and prescribed drugs have certain contraindications and potential side effects, and may or may not help you to achieve an acceptable level of pain relief. Medications which act purely as analgesics do nothing whatsoever to impact on the underlying cause of the problem and so only really mask the pain, and a safe return to former levels of mobility is highly unlikely if drugs are used in isolation. Patients are either inclined to continue life at their current levels of mobility without ever seeing any improvement (and whilst often experiencing further deterioration) or, if the pain is wholly eliminated, can be tempted to overdo things and make their conditions worse.

Another problem with relying solely on medicinal treatments in cases of neck and back, and indeed any other type of chronic pain, is that in many cases the effects of the drugs lessen over time. While it may be possible in the early days to increase dosages to make the pain more bearable, obviously there comes a point where the body's maximum tolerance level is reached and it would be unsafe to do so any further. As the tolerance to one particular drug can sometimes mean tolerance to all of the others within the same group of medicines, the options in terms of medication can eventually become limited or exhausted and pain levels can begin to soar anew. It is hardly surprising, therefore, that patients who suffer from chronic pain conditions are at the highest risk of self-medicating, whether by taking excessive doses of prescribed medications or by turning to alcohol or illicit drugs.

Of course, eliminating or reducing pain is an extremely important starting point if you are suffering from a problem with either the neck or back, because without doing so, any further treatment which is designed to bring about improvement in the condition can feel impossible. It is, however, just that ... a starting point and a foundation on which long-lasting relief and dramatic improvements to quality of life can be built.

As human beings, most of us have short memories when it comes to unpleasant experiences, so that when pain subsides we forget just how bad it made us feel, not just physically, but emotionally and psychologically too. We simply take the painkillers or the anti-inflammatories, feel at least partially better and put the episode behind us. Now, while this might work in some cases, such as if we have broken a toe and there is little if anything of worth that the medical profession can do, in the main it is a pretty risky strategy. Taking antibiotics and analgesics to get rid of an abscess underneath a tooth might solve the problem in the short term, but unless we attend to the broken filling or whatever was responsible for causing the abscess in the first place, the problem will not only return, but is likely to return more quickly and get worse each time.

In the case of conditions which affect the neck and back, the same principle is true. While painkillers might mask the pain and allow you to go about your daily activities, if you continue to use your body in ways which put undue pressure and strain on the affected area, then you will be doomed to taking increasing doses throughout your life as your condition continues to worsen. If you take anti-inflammatory drugs until the inflammation subsides but do nothing to work on improving mobility, gait or posture, then again the inflammation is likely to return.

As I have already described, by far the most effective way of tackling conditions which cause pain to the neck or back is by taking a holistic and multidisciplinary approach to treatment and, in this, physiotherapy plays a huge and immensely important role. Although most people's perception of physiotherapy is of being put through rigorous and painful exercises in an attempt to restore them to full functionality, in fact, this is not only an inaccurate reflection on the role of physiotherapists, but also a very incomplete one.

The formal definition of physiotherapy as quoted in the Chartered Society of Physiotherapy's 2002 Curriculum Framework is as follows:

> *It uses physical approaches to promote, maintain and restore physical, psychological and social well-being, taking account of variations in health status. Physiotherapy is science-based, committed to extending, applying, evaluating and reviewing the evidence that underpins and informs its practice and delivery. The exercise of clinical judgement and informed interpretation is at its core.*

As you can see, far from being about bending the body into impossible shapes and positions, physiotherapy is aimed at restoring movement and function to as near normal as possible so that the patient's well-being and quality of life are positively impacted at all levels. The techniques which are used to achieve this, while they do include exercise, are in fact very wide ranging and encompass everything from education to a whole variety of specialised treatments.

Thankfully, the world of medicine never stands still and alongside the more traditional treatments for neck and back pain, a whole raft of new ones is constantly being developed. While it may take both time and more evidence of their effectiveness for some or all of these to be accepted by organisations such as the National Institute for Health and Clinical Excellence (NICE), in the meantime many are proving to offer significant relief to a great many people.

Of course, regardless of whether treatments are traditional and widely accepted or considered by some to be more controversial, pain is a very subjective thing and every person reacts differently to different methods. As we look at some of the ancient and more modern techniques which are employed by physiotherapists today, therefore, it is worth bearing in mind that although NICE may consider that there is insufficient evidence for them to be able to recommend some of the more recent innovations as being effective, there are also other well-respected clinical organisations which still dispute the effectiveness of treatments such as acupuncture which have been around for centuries and have brought immense amounts of pain relief to millions of sufferers.

Even if you personally have reservations about some of the techniques described in the remainder of this chapter, it is my hope that you will at least have a better understanding of what medicine and science have to offer and so be able to make better and more well-informed decisions in terms of your treatment.

Education

In deciding to read this book, you have of course started down the road of self-education, but the role of the trained physiotherapist is one which takes education to an entirely different level. While in a book such as this it is entirely possible to talk in broader terms, what cannot be done is to evaluate or address the unique aspects of each individual's condition or circumstances. This, however, is precisely what your own physiotherapist can do.

As well as that in relation to exercises which are designed specifically to help your particular condition or injury, the type of education that you can expect to receive might include:

- how to carry out your normal day-to-day activities as normally and as safely as possible;
- how to protect and avoid further injury to your neck or back;
- how to protect and avoid injury to other parts of the body which may be affected by guarding or altered gait or posture;
- how to sit, stand and walk so as not to aggravate or worsen your condition;
- how to make adjustments in your home and workplace to make life easier and avoid further deterioration to your condition;
- how to use equipment such as back braces or apply treatments such as cold, ice or heat treatments at home;
- how to choose furniture such as beds and chairs which will help to improve your posture.

Manual therapy

Manual therapy, which as the name suggests involves treatment applied with the hands, can take a number of forms which might be aimed at reducing pain, increasing flexibility and mobility or promoting relaxation. It is important to note that some or all of these therapies may not be appropriate for certain neck or back conditions, however, and that all should only be undertaken if recommended by a qualified medical practitioner and carried out by a fully trained and qualified therapist.

Massage is probably the most well-known form of manual therapy and, although it does not help to strengthen the neck or back or make them more flexible, it can be very beneficial in terms of easing pain, improving circulation and removing tension from the muscles. The pressure which is used in therapeutic massage is generally only mild, but of course it is still vital that it only be performed by a physiotherapist who is not only trained and experienced in treating neck and back conditions, but also fully aware of your medical history, so that further damage or injury is not incurred.

Mobilisation, as the name suggests, is a technique which is aimed at overcoming stiffness and increasing the range of motion by overcoming restrictions such as in joints, muscles, tendons or ligaments which might have been strained, for example as the result of a whiplash-type injury, or which might even have been deliberately immobilised in order to minimise the effects of pain. Starting gently, the therapist will gradually increase pressure and encourage greater range of movement as the patient begins to move with less discomfort.

The third main type of manual therapy is manipulation, which is typically used to help reposition bones and joints. In order to achieve its aims, it is by necessity quite a forceful type of therapy involving a high-velocity thrust technique which is by no means suitable for all types of neck and back conditions. In fact, there have been reported cases of manipulation being the cause of herniated discs, vertebral fractures, spinal cord compression and nerve root compression, so it is always advisable to discuss the benefits and risks of this treatment with your physiotherapist before going ahead.

Cold and ice treatments

Another very useful type of treatment which may be recommended by physiotherapists is that which uses either cold or ice packs to provide relief from the pain and swelling which often accompany injuries to the neck or back, such as strains and sprains which often cause muscle spasms and stiffness, as well as neck and back disorders. These simple but effective treatments work to:

■ slow down and minimise swelling and inflammation after injury, so reducing pain;

■ numb tissues by acting as a local anaesthetic;

■ decrease muscle spasms;

■ decrease the extent of tissue damage;

■ make the veins contract, so that when the cold is removed and the veins dilate again, blood, which is full of all the nutrients that the body needs to heal itself, rushes back into the area;

■ affect the nerve impulses, so interrupting pain messages.

Although cold or ice treatments might appear to be harmless, care does still need to be taken to avoid 'burns' to the skin or the restriction of blood circulation. Always be sure to follow your therapist's directions when using cold or ice packs at home and remember to place a protective barrier between ice and the skin and limit the ice application to no more than 15 or 20 minutes. In addition, it is important not to use ice therapy before taking part in any kind of strenuous activity, because this will cause the muscles and the blood vessels to constrict, which could lead to further injury.

Cold or ice therapy may not be suitable for all types of neck and back conditions and those who suffer from rheumatoid arthritis and certain other conditions should therefore avoid its use. In cases where there are no contraindications, cold or ice treatments are typically combined with other types of therapies and treatments to provide maximum pain-relieving effect.

Heat treatments

In the same way that cold and ice therapy can help to reduce swelling and inflammation, especially in the immediate aftermath of an injury, applying heat soon afterwards can actually cause the affected area to swell and so should be avoided for at least a couple of days. Thereafter, however, heat therapy can provide a number of benefits to sufferers of either acute or chronic neck or back pain by:

- dilating the blood vessels and improving blood circulation so that the flow of oxygen and nutrients to the injured area is increased, healing promoted and painful muscle spasms relieved;
- stimulating the sensory receptors in the skin, which has the effect of reducing the transmission of pain signals to the brain;
- allowing the soft tissues around the spine to stretch so that stiffness is eased and flexibility increased.

As with cold and ice therapy, care must be taken with heat treatments to ensure that the skin is not burned and so again, a towel or something similar should be placed between the source of the heat and the skin. Applications should again be limited, with 20 to 30 minutes being the maximum time per session.

Heat can be applied to the back or neck in a number of different ways to achieve relief from pain. Hot water bottles, special heat packs, wraps or compresses, hot, moist towels or even a hot bath can do much to improve comfort levels, and of course for those who wish to use heat therapy at home, at work or whilst travelling, for example, many of these solutions are not only very inexpensive, but highly practical too. It is also worth remembering that heat therapy is not just useful in terms of providing pain relief and increasing mobility, but also helps to relax and warm the muscles before exercising, which is vital if further injury is to be avoided.

Again as with cold and ice therapy, heat therapy tends to work best when it is combined with other treatment techniques such as manual therapy and exercise, and of course it represents an appealing alternative to many patients who prefer to avoid pharmaceutical drugs.

Hydrotherapy

Hydrotherapy treatments have been used in a variety of forms for centuries and whether these involve being totally immersed in water or simply sitting in a steam room, they have the potential to help heal the body and reduce pain, as well as making exercise much more bearable. Whirlpools, Jacuzzis, water spas, saunas, steam rooms, swimming pools and even your own bath tub are all forms of hydrotherapy. Studies have shown that people who soak in a warm bath not only experience less stiffness and greater flexibility, but also tend to use less pain medication.

Depending on the temperature of the water, hydrotherapy works in much the same way as ice and cold and heat treatments in that it increases or restricts blood circulation and impacts on the transmission of pain signals. In addition, however, when immersed in water, the body is relieved of the force of gravity which is normally exerted, so taking any of the usual pressure off painful joints and muscles as well as providing gentle resistance which helps to build strength and flexibility. Hydrotherapy has proved to be particularly useful for those suffering with chronic lower back pain, but it is important that water exercise therapy is supervised by a qualified physiotherapist to ensure that no further damage or injury is sustained.

Although hydrotherapy is safe for most sufferers of neck and back pain, diabetics and those who are sensitive to temperature do need to take particular care. In addition, pregnant women should avoid the use of saunas.

Acupuncture

Although there are those who dispute the effectiveness of acupuncture in terms of its ability to reduce pain, a great many people do find that it has tremendous effect. Those in the medical field who do have faith in its healing and painkilling powers, meanwhile, are divided as to quite how it works, with some believing that it affects the flow of the body's vital energy or life force and others attributing its effects to scientific and biological changes.

As many will know, acupuncture involves the placing of very fine needles into specific points on the skin. Although this sounds, and to some people looks painful, in fact it is rare for anything more than slight discomfort or a mild tingling sensation to be felt and the experience certainly bears no comparison with receiving an injection. While those who accept the more traditional Chinese beliefs assert that the treatment corrects or maintains the normal flow of qi (the life force), a more scientific explanation might be that the insertion of the needle provokes a chemical or electrical response in the body which allows pain-relieving hormones to be released and muscles to relax.

The number of acupuncture needles used by the specialist varies from patient to patient and according to the nature and severity of the condition, but is normally anything up to around 20. In some cases these may do nothing more than just break the surface of the skin, but where deeper layers of muscle need to be reached, longer needles of up to nine inches in length may be required. Often, once inserted they will be left in the body for 15–30 minutes, and they may be turned in one direction or the other, but in some cases they will be inserted and removed after just a matter of seconds. Some types of acupuncture treatment also use needles which are warmed or charged electrically after insertion.

As with any type of therapeutic treatment, it is absolutely vital that acupuncture is only delivered by a trained and qualified specialist of high reputation, particularly because of the dangers associated with the use of needles. Practitioners should only use single-use, disposable needles which are kept in sterile packaging to ensure the safety of patients.

Acupressure

Rather than using needles, the treatment known as acupressure relies on the practitioner's fingers to apply gentle pressure to strategic parts of the body known as acupoints, which may or may not be located at or close to the source of the pain. As with acupuncture, the origin of this type of treatment goes back thousands of years and is based on the belief that blocked energy which leads to both physical and emotional pain and discomfort can be released by manipulating certain points on the body to allow the body's life force to flow freely and balance the body's natural energies.

Acupressure is another treatment which draws scepticism from some within the field of medicine. Although there is no scientific evidence to support the theories upon which acupressure are based, however, some studies have suggested that the application of pressure to certain points on the body causes the brain to release more endorphins, the body's natural painkillers. Whether or not the theories are proven though, many people experience considerable relief from pain and tense muscles as a result of this type of therapy and so it offers another valuable alternative or addition to more traditional forms of treatment.

Exercise

What comes to mind when most people think about physiotherapy is exercise, and although it is of course only one of a range of tools that the therapist has at his or her disposal to help those with neck and back problems, it is nevertheless a very important one.

It goes without saying that everyone benefits from being physically fit, but for anyone who suffers from neck or back pain, whether acute or chronic, it can not only feel difficult, but even impossible to carry out just the most ordinary of movements, let alone anything more vigorous. Excruciating pain, coupled with stiffness, typically leads to the loss of normal function as the muscles and joints in the body lose their strength and flexibility, and without exercise, the result can be permanent mobility problems or even complete disability.

The range of exercises used by physiotherapists is vast, but in every case the ones which are selected are designed to match the unique requirements and capabilities of the individual patient. Accurate diagnosis of the person's condition is, of course, vital in ensuring that the exercise regime proposed is appropriate, and education in terms of how the exercises should be performed is crucial too, in order that no further injury or damage results from the prescribed activities. Exercises are designed to start slow and build up gradually in intensity as pain levels and flexibility improve through the exercises themselves, as well as through the other pharmaceutical and non-pharmaceutical treatments which form part of the multidisciplinary treatment package.

As every case of neck and back pain is different, it is of course impossible to generalise in terms of the types of activities which may be prescribed, but stretching exercises and those which are aimed at strengthening the muscles, such as through the use of weights, often form part of a typical exercise regime. Walking, swimming, aerobic exercises and activities such as yoga, however, can also be highly beneficial. Before embarking on any kind of exercise activity though, it is important that you seek the advice of your therapist to ensure that there are no medical considerations which would make it inadvisable and that your approach to the exercise programme is appropriate and safe.

In those who are at the peak of fitness, as well as those who suffer from injuries, diseases and disorders, exercise plays a huge role in ensuring psychological as well as physical well-being. The hormones which are released during exercise do not just reduce pain and promote healing, but they also provide an overall sense of well-being. As there is quite often a psychological component to chronic neck and back pain conditions, exercise in fact performs a triple role in terms of restoring patients to physical, mental and emotional health.

Although physiotherapists work with their patients to teach them the exercises which form part of their programmes and some activities will be carried out with their direct supervision, the importance of continuing the exercises at home cannot be stressed strongly enough. For function and mobility to be restored to as normal levels as possible, and in order that further pain, injury and degeneration of the spine are to be avoided, it is vital that they be carried out on a regular basis so that tissues and muscles are taught to behave in a different and healthier way through repetition. Set yourself specific times throughout the day to carry out your exercises to ensure that you maintain the momentum because, unlike some other types of treatment, exercise is not likely to yield any immediate results. Only by sticking rigorously to your exercise programme will you truly obtain long-lasting, overall benefits.

Posture

Poor posture is not only responsible for aggravating neck and back problems, but in some cases it actually causes them to develop in the first place. How you sit, stand and lie down, although these are things which most of us do not give much conscious thought to, can have an enormous, if not necessarily positive, impact on the spine, and so these are other areas in which a trained and qualified physiotherapist can provide hugely valuable support and advice.

Our posture, or the way that we hold our bodies upright against the force of gravity, of course changes according to what we are doing. Whether we are standing up, walking, bending, lifting, sitting or lying down, however, there are optimum ways of doing so which avoid too much strain being placed on the muscles, joints and ligaments and which ensure that the spine remains properly aligned. In fact, developing and maintaining good posture has a range of benefits, such as:

- ensuring that bones and joints are aligned correctly so that muscles are used more efficiently and in a balanced way;
- reducing any abnormal wear and tear on the surfaces of the joints which could result in arthritis;
- reducing the stress on the ligaments which hold the joints of the spine together;
- ensuring the even distribution of weight;
- allowing the muscles to be used more efficiently, so preventing fatigue;
- preventing the spine from becoming fixed in abnormal positions;
- ensuring that the vital organs are in the right positions and able to function at peak efficiency;
- minimising the potential for strain or overuse of joints and muscles;
- preventing back, neck and muscular pain.

In some cases, an accident or injury can cause the development of poor posture as the patient adapts the way that he or she sits, stands, moves or lies in order to avoid pain, but in other cases it results simply from bad habits. Whatever the reason, however, slouching and slumping causes the spine to become misaligned so that the natural curves in the neck and back become distorted. Over time, this causes changes in the way that muscles and ligaments behave and very often leads to pain and stiffness, not to mention changes in the body's appearance. By teaching you how to control your posture, a physiotherapist can help you to use your spine and muscles efficiently, with the least amount of muscle activity, so that valuable energy is not expended in everyday movements.

As with exercise, it is vital that posture is not just something that you think about when visiting the physiotherapist. If positive changes in the condition of the back and neck are to be brought about and maintained, good postural habits need to be reinforced at all times, whether you are at home, at work, driving in your car or in any other situation. In the following chapter on self-help, you will find some general guidelines on how to improve posture, but as your physiotherapist will be fully *au fait* with your condition and your medical history, it is important to note that any advice that he or she provides should be given precedence over these.

Low-level laser therapy

Low-level laser therapy (LLLT) is used in the treatment of humans, as well as in veterinary treatment. It uses low-level lasers to reduce inflammation and encourage tissue repair by altering cell function. Although research is still ongoing in terms of whether it works best when used over the nerves or the joints, as well as to establish the optimum wavelength, pulsing, dose, timing and duration, several studies have already shown it to be effective in 70% of patients who were suffering from acute neck pain, even though the pain could not be linked to a specific cause. In these cases, reduced levels of pain were experienced immediately after the treatment had been applied. Those with chronic neck pain also benefitted from LLLT, although generally it seems to take longer (up to 22 weeks in some cases) for the effects to be felt.

LLLT cannot only be used to treat neck pain and reports suggest that it also provides effective relief from short-term back pain caused by osteoarthritis and rheumatoid arthritis.

Therapeutic ultrasound

Therapeutic ultrasound uses very high frequency sound waves to stimulate the tissue up to 12.7 cm below the skin's surface in what might be described as a high frequency massage. The heating and massaging effects increase blood flow, which in turn speeds up the healing process, as well as reducing swelling and oedema (swelling caused by fluid retention) which can often be the source of pain, particularly when an injury to the neck or back has been sustained.

For maximum benefit, it is suggested that therapeutic ultrasound treatments be carried out for 5–10 minutes, 2–3 times per day throughout the duration of the healing period.

Interferential current therapy

Interferential current therapy (IFC) is an electrotherapeutic technique which has not, in fact, only recently come into use but has been around since the 1950s. Used to treat a range of chronic conditions including sciatica, chronic neck and lower back pain and osteoarthritis, it involves passing a medium frequency electrical current through the back or neck with the aims of accelerating healing whilst at the same time stimulating the production of the body's natural painkillers, endorphins. Many who have tried it report not only immediate, but also long-lasting pain relief and, like therapeutic ultrasound, it can also be very effective at increasing local blood flow and reducing swelling and oedema.

Transcutaneous electrical nerve stimulation

Transcutaneous electrical nerve stimulation, or TENS as it is more commonly known, is a technique which delivers small, high or low frequency electrical pulses via electrodes which are connected to the skin. Used at high frequencies, it is believed to selectively stimulate certain nerve fibres which are not responsible for carrying pain messages, so that these send signals which effectively block other nerve signals which are carrying pain messages. At low frequencies, meanwhile, the device is thought to stimulate the production of endorphins, the body's natural painkillers, although it is not suitable for:

- those who suffer from epilepsy;
- people who suffer from certain types of heart disease;
- those who have pacemakers fitted;
- people whose cause of pain is unknown;
- women who are considering using it unsupervised during pregnancy (except during labour).

TENS is generally considered to be safe and appears to have few side effects. Although traditionally used by women during labour, it is now commonly used by many women to help them cope with menstrual pains and is widely marketed for musculoskeletal pain relief.

Case Study 3

A 64-year-old man attended the London Pain Clinic complaining of pain in the L3/4 area of his lumbar spine and an aching, deep-seated pain. He had been experiencing the pain for the last six years, but stated that it had increased in frequency over the last three months. The pain, which was only occasionally relieved by a combination of paracetamol and dihydrocodeine (opioid painkillers), was aggravated by exercise and he was unable to walk further than 50 yards without being in extreme discomfort.

When the gentleman first came to the clinic, he was taking Remedeine 2 tablets 1–4 times a day (containing paracetamol 500 mg and dihydrocodeine 30 mg), as well as the antidepressants Cipralex 10 mg and amitriptyline 20 mg and the benzodiazepine Diazepam. His past medical history indicated no stomach or peptic ulceration, but intermittent episodes of diarrhoea as well as depression, but no other medical problems. He had previously been given a diagnosis of reactive depression and was under the care of a psychiatrist for this. When his depression was discussed with the patient and his wife, it was revealed that he had suffered severe bouts, but with the help of the medication had been able to start functioning and interacting socially once again.

Further investigation revealed that the gentleman had experienced a crushed fracture in the thoracic region of the back in 1999, and a prolapsed disc to the L4/5 lumbar vertebrae. The disc prolapse had been serious in nature and, because of the incapacitation that it had caused him, he had a discectomy operation to correct it.

During examination it was noted that the gentleman had a marked kyphosis (forward curvature of the spine). His original height had been 1.91 m and he felt that he had lost at least 5 cm in height. On palpation, there was a reduction in flexion/extension and lateral movement of the lumbar spine. Although no facet joint tenderness was evident at any level, there was left sacroiliac joint tenderness on deep palpation. Overall, there was reduced lower limb power and the patient walked with a stick. The patient was diagnosed with osteoarthritis of the lower lumbar spine with co-existing osteoporosis.

The treatment plan which was recommended for the gentleman included the prescription of Diclofenac 75 mg slow release (a non-steroidal anti-inflammatory drug) twice a day and co-dydramol (a compound analgesic) as required and he was also put on an intensive course of outpatient physiotherapy. We also discussed with the psychiatrist the possibility of adjusting the doses of his medication, in particular the Cipralex, amitriptyline and Diazepam. As the patient was already using mild opiates and suffering from a stiff and painful back and these additional medications were causing shaking and unsteadiness on the feet, it was felt that these treatments were increasing his potential for falls.

The medication was duly adjusted and the gentleman underwent six sessions of physiotherapy. Gentle exercises were carried out during the sessions, but the patient also continued with these on a daily basis at home. Although he found that the pain was immediately worse after physiotherapy, it then greatly improved and so he started taking his 'as required' analgesic medication in order to get him through these episodes. At the final consultation following his six physiotherapy sessions, he had made an impressive and dramatic improvement in terms of the levels of pain that he experienced. In addition, he was significantly more flexible and was experiencing fewer adverse effects on the lower doses of medication that he had been prescribed. The gentleman was then discharged from the clinic.

11

Self-Help and Herbal Medicines

As you will have seen in the preceding chapters, there is much that the medical profession can do to help patients with painful neck and back injuries and conditions to experience less discomfort and a vastly improved quality of life. As I said earlier, however, our memories can sometimes be short and once some relief from pain and stiffness has been achieved through, for example pharmaceutical drugs and/or manual therapies, it can be tempting for patients to relax their efforts and return to old habits. If long-lasting improvements are to be achieved though, it is vital that sufferers take the initiative in terms of self-help and in the remainder of this chapter you will find some useful tips which are aimed at helping you to do just that.

In Chapter 9, I outlined some of the main pharmaceutical drugs which are used in the treatment of neck and back conditions and how these work, but of course there is also a range of herbal medications which many people find to be highly effective. Towards the end of this chapter, you will also find information concerning some of those which are most commonly used and reported to be most beneficial.

Rest and activity

When neck and back pain strike, many people's first reaction is to lie down and rest in order to alleviate the symptoms. Research has demonstrated quite clearly, however, that bed rest for more than two days is not good for the back. Although it might appear to offer some temporary relief, in the longer term it causes greater inflexibility and immobility and increased rather than decreased levels of pain.

While over-the-counter and prescribed medications can do much to alleviate pain and stiffness, sometimes their effect is only partial and/or temporary and patients may be left with residual symptoms.

Often though, the expectations of drug treatments are unreasonably high and sufferers wait indefinitely for them to render them completely free of pain and stiffness before trying to embark on their normal activities. In fact though, not only is it unnecessary to wait until you are totally pain-free, but it can often exacerbate the problem.

Of course, in cases where pain and stiffness are severe, it is highly unlikely that you will be able to undertake the same level of activity as you could previously. If this is the case, then try to pace yourself by doing less or doing things at a slower rate and gradually do a little more each day. Unless it is specifically recommended by an expert in neck and back conditions who is familiar with the history and nature of your condition, however, do not refrain from normal activities and resort to extended bed rest.

Another thing to be careful of is sitting or standing for prolonged periods of time. Whether you are working at a computer, watching the television or whatever, make sure that you get up and move around every half hour or so to avoid the body becoming stiff and sore. If necessary, set yourself an alarm to remind you.

Working life

While there may be special circumstances to take into account in relation to your working environment, generally it is not advisable to delay a return to work after an absence caused by a neck or back pain injury or disorder until you are entirely pain-free. Not only will going to work each day help you to remain physically active and so help in terms of regaining normal levels of mobility, but it also helps to provide a sense of normality in your life and can work as an effective distraction from your symptoms.

If your work involves heavy lifting or carrying, then it is important to discuss this with your physician to find out whether it is safe for you to continue and, if so, to receive expert advice on how you can best avoid any aggravation to your condition or any recurrence of the problem. Even in jobs which are largely sedentary by nature, however, there may still be certain adjustments, such as to your workstation, which may need to be made to ensure that you are able to work safely and comfortably. Nowadays, many employers have their own in-house Health and Safety representatives who will be able to carry out a workplace assessment and recommend any beneficial changes or equipment, so be sure to seek their help.

Another thing which is worth considering if, for example, your symptoms feel worse at a particular time of day, is a change to your former working patterns. Working flexible rather than fixed hours might allow you to attend work during those hours when you feel at your best and are less distracted by pain, while working at home for some of the time might help if you have a long commute to contend with or when bad weather conditions present additional risks of slipping or falling. Largely because of the changes which have come about due to advances in modern technology, many employers today are much more open to revised working arrangements such as these, so do not be afraid to discuss the possibility if you think that it might help.

The alternative of giving up work altogether, although it might at first seem appealing, can see people becoming extremely isolated, depressed and inactive, not to mention being more conscious of their pain and causing additional worries and stresses with respect to their financial situations. So do what you can to continue with your normal occupation, even if this does mean having to make a few changes to your working arrangements.

Retaining a positive mental attitude

Research indicates that those who retain a positive mental attitude in the face of serious illness and chronic pain conditions fare much better in a physical, emotional and psychological sense than those who do not. Their bodies heal more quickly and efficiently and their symptoms tend to be much less severe.

Discovering that you are suffering from a chronic pain condition which may never be fully resolved is undoubtedly a frightening experience. Sufferers often find themselves thinking in terms of worse case scenarios, not just in respect of their own lives, but also in relation to how their relationships with their partners, children, family members and friends will be affected, and their working lives. All of these gloomy thoughts and predictions, however, simply increase stress and tension and exacerbate the problem, and the reality in terms of neck and back conditions is that rarely are these serious or life-threatening. Always be sure to visit a reputable physician who specialises in dealing with neck and back conditions and can diagnose your condition accurately, as this will not only ensure that you receive the appropriate treatment, but also stop your mind from running riot and imagining that things are worse than they really are.

Depending upon the nature and extent of the neck or back condition, the fact is that you may have to make certain adjustments to your former way of life, but this in no way means that your quality of life need suffer. Indeed, many people who have managed to retain a positive mental attitude towards their conditions have found that it has caused them to take up activities which they might never have considered before and meet people whom they might not otherwise have met.

Not just in terms of health, life has a habit of throwing the unexpected our way, but what matters is how we choose to respond to these events – and we do have a choice. By recognising and adjusting negative thought patterns, the human mind can be retrained to think in a positive way. If you find that you are struggling to achieve this on your own, there are numerous self-help books available online or at local bookstores which walk the reader step by step through the process.

Following recommendations

As I have mentioned on a number of occasions throughout the course of this book, a multidisciplinary approach to treating neck and back pain has proven time and time again to be the most effective. Working alongside a trained, qualified and experienced pain management specialist, you will have a comprehensive and unique package of treatments which is designed to ensure maximum relief from symptoms and the very best quality of life. Clearly, for this combination of treatments to work as intended though, requires that the specialist's recommendations are followed and that you play an active role in keeping him or her up to date with any adverse effects that any aspect of treatment might be having.

The first area to mention in terms of recommendations is regarding medication, whether that be over-the-counter or prescribed. Even if you know other sufferers who are taking higher or lower dosages of certain drugs, it is never appropriate for you to adjust your own and in fact it could prove highly dangerous for you to do so. Your specialist will have prescribed your medication so that it takes into account the nature and extent of your condition, any co-existing illnesses or disorders, your family history, your tolerance to certain drugs, any allergies that you might suffer from and a whole host of other considerations, and what is appropriate for others may be totally inappropriate for you.

If you find that certain drugs are having little or no impact on your symptoms or that they are causing distressing side effects, then discuss these matters directly with your physician before making any changes and under no circumstances consider self-medication using prescribed medication, alcohol or illicit drugs. Even if you are using over-the-counter preparations, either as an alternative to or in conjunction with prescribed medications, always check with your doctor or the pharmacist to ensure that there are no contraindications.

With regard to the various types of therapies which might be recommended, again any reputable specialist will only prescribe what he or she considers to be beneficial and appropriate for your particular circumstances to bring about maximum relief. If therapy sessions are prescribed with a particular degree of regularity, then be sure that you do not miss appointments, even if you do not see immediate results. Some types of therapy, such as exercise therapy, take time for their effects to be felt, but it is still essential that you keep up with the recommended activities at the prescribed level of intensity. Train yourself to do precisely what has been recommended rather than overdoing things on good days and possibly setting yourself back, or under-doing them on bad days. If you have any fears concerning the effectiveness of any of your treatments, then discuss these with your specialist so that you fully understand the reasons why they have been prescribed and so that any adjustments to your treatment programme can be made if required.

Recommendations concerning posture, specialist equipment or even basic furniture for use at home or in the workplace are also offered for your direct benefit and so every effort should be made to follow these if you are to experience speedy recovery, maximum relief from symptoms and the return to an acceptable quality of life.

Setting goals

While it might be easy to carry on taking prescribed medications, keeping yourself motivated to continue with exercise programmes or just continue with normal daily activities can become difficult when you are suffering from chronic pain. Progress may at times feel slow and there may sometimes be the temptation to just give up altogether.

One way to try and overcome these feelings is to set yourself a series of goals, not just in relation to improving your physical condition, but in relation to other aspects of your life too. If your condition has caused you to restrict your social activities for instance, then set yourself a goal which ensures that you meet up with friends or family members once a week regardless of how you are feeling. As you meet and surpass each of these goals, your sense of accomplishment and determination will grow and your situation will soon begin to feel much less hopeless than you could have imagined because you will feel in control of your own life, rather than having your condition dictate it for you.

Talking

We have all heard the old saying 'A problem shared is a problem halved', and while it is important to avoid talking incessantly or whingeing and whining about your pain and other symptoms, it is equally important that the people in your life understand your problem, your treatment and the things that you are doing to help yourself. In addition, you need to be able to ask for help when this is necessary.

Some of the reasons for talking to other people are practical ones. If you are taking medications which have the effect of impairing your abilities or have the potential to cause dangerous or distressing side effects, for example, then it is advisable that others are aware of this. If your working life is likely to be affected by your condition or adjustments need to be made to your working environment, then clearly you will want to communicate these things to your employer.

Talking, however, is not just about dealing with practicalities, but also about dealing with difficult feelings and emotions.

Living with a chronic pain condition often raises all kinds of fears such as whether you might become permanently disabled or whether partners or friends will still want you in their lives when you can, at least temporarily, no longer take part in the activities that you used to share. Bottling these fears up and not talking about them not only means that you are working on speculation without knowing whether there is any basis to them, but also that misunderstandings can arise, that fears can grow out of all proportion, that you are robbed of the opportunity to be understood and supported and that others are equally robbed of the chance to offer the help that most would dearly like to give.

Try to discuss your fears, concerns and insecurities in a matter-of-fact way which simply describes them rather than being designed to elicit pity. Those who are worthy of being a part of your life will want to understand and to be able to support you appropriately, so be sure to keep the communication lines open.

Reducing stress

As we saw back in Chapter 6, stress can have an enormous impact in an emotional, psychological and physical sense. Even a person who is physically fit and healthy but suffers from stress will soon begin to experience very real and sometimes disturbing bouts of pain in unexpected parts of the body. There are otherwise healthy women, for instance, who have been rushed into hospital for emergency exploratory operations for suspected ectopic pregnancies, whose pain was actually caused solely and directly by stress. Although it might be hard to believe that the human body could react in such an extreme way as this, in fact cases such as these are not uncommon and symptoms can be frighteningly similar to those of an array of much more serious complaints.

If stress on its own can cause such a high degree of discomfort in otherwise healthy individuals, it is not hard to see what impact it might have on those who are already in pain. The muscle tension caused by stress is notorious for affecting the neck and back, and coupled with the pain from the original injury or condition, it can become excruciating. Identifying and then either avoiding stressful situations or people or reducing the impact of stress is therefore vital if symptoms are not to be exacerbated and the quality of life improved.

In such a stress-ridden society as ours, there have been numerous excellent books written about the subject and there are numerous techniques that you can try to help alleviate its effects. Some of these work better for certain individuals than they do for others, so if you find that some have little or no effect, do not force them or allow them to stress you out further, but simply try something different. Here are some suggestions that you might like to consider to help you to relax:

- meditation;
- physical relaxation and therapies such as breathing exercises, yoga or massage;
- relaxation tapes;
- music therapy;
- immersing yourself in activities that you enjoy;
- taking up a creative hobby;
- writing;
- relaxing in a warm bath;
- watching a favourite comedy programme or movie;
- taking a quiet walk on your own or taking time out in a quiet space.

Sometimes, dealing with stress requires some much more fundamental changes in life. Although you may not have been used to planning and scheduling your time in the past or living with a routine, knowing what is around the corner and ensuring greater predictability in your life can be a highly effective way of minimising those nasty surprises which cause stress. Facing problems head-on, rather than avoiding them and letting them play on your mind, can also lead to much greater peace of mind, simply because this allows you to feel in greater control of your life. You do not have to deal with them all at once if that would feel overwhelming, but just take them one at a time so that little by little your stress levels reduce. Talk to the bank manager, initiate that difficult relationship conversation with your partner or have that heart to heart with your boss; at least then you will stand a chance of finding a resolution and being able to sleep at night.

Another couple of things which are well worth working at are becoming more assertive and learning to ask for help. Women in particular often find it hard to say 'no' without feeling immensely guilty and so even though they might be suffering themselves, can still take on too much and suffer stress when they begin to find things overwhelming. Both men and women, meanwhile, can have difficulties in asking for the help that they need, although often others are only too happy to do what they can to assist.

Not surprisingly, we all build up certain expectations of ourselves as we go through life and learn what we are capable of. Unfortunately though, even when situations and circumstances change, it can be hard to let these go. If you are suffering from pain and restrictions to mobility, it is however unreasonable to expect yourself to be able to operate at the same level, so think carefully about what you can realistically achieve and then revise your expectations accordingly.

Addressing weight issues

If you are suffering from serious weight issues alongside a neck or back condition, this may be something which is raised by your healthcare specialist who may recommend a weight loss diet. Even without neck and back problems, carrying excess weight is damaging to overall health and well-being and can cause heart disease and a whole range of other conditions. The extra pressure which is exerted on bones, joints and muscles, however, can also add to the levels of pain and discomfort for anyone with a neck or back injury or disorder, and being overweight is likely to further restrict mobility.

Even in those who do not normally suffer from problems with weight, chronic pain conditions can represent a challenge when pain and stiffness impact on normal levels of activity. Foods which might not have caused weight gain in the past when you were rushing around burning up calories might begin to 'stick to the hips' and so it may be useful to keep an eye on the scales and take action with respect to diet before things start to get out of hand.

Although books and websites promote a bewildering array of weight loss diets, it has to be said that not all of these are necessarily considered to be either safe or healthy. At any time, the human body requires certain nutrients to ensure that it functions well, and of course when it is trying to recover from illness or injury, these are all the more essential. Before committing yourself to any weight reduction plan, therefore, always seek the advice of your healthcare provider to satisfy yourself that it is appropriate and safe.

Posture

Developing and maintaining good postural habits is essential if the effects of existing neck and back problems are to be minimised and further problems avoided. Posture may be an issue which is covered by your physiotherapist and you may be given specific guidance to follow as part of your overall treatment programme, but to follow you will find some general guidelines for safer sitting, standing, driving, lifting and handling and lying down or sleeping.

Sitting
- Choose an upright chair with good back support and avoid those which are low or soft.
- Sit with your back straight, your shoulders back and your buttocks touching the back of the chair.
- If necessary, use a small cushion, a rolled-up towel or a lumbar roll to support the small of the back and maintain the spine's natural curves.
- Keep your knees and hips level or your knees slightly higher than your hips and use a footrest or stool if necessary.
- Do not cross your legs or ankles but keep your feet flat on the floor.
- Make sure that your body weight is evenly distributed on both hips.
- When rising from a seated position, move to the front of the chair seat and stand up by straightening your legs rather than bending forward at the waist.
- Avoid sitting in the same position for more than 20 or 30 minutes at a time and set yourself an alarm if necessary to remind you to get up and move around.
- When working at a computer, make sure that the height of your chair and workstation are adjusted so that you are able to sit up close to your work. Your forearms should be horizontal to the desk or keyboard, your elbows at right angles and your shoulders relaxed.
- Make sure that your head is positioned centrally to your spine and to the computer screen and that your screen is at eye level. Also, use a

copy holder for any reference materials and make sure this too is at eye level and close to the screen.

- If you use a chair which rolls or pivots, turn your whole body while sitting rather than twisting at the waist.

Standing

- Wear comfortable shoes with low heels and cushioned soles as these will help to reduce the stress on the back.
- Stand upright with your head facing forwards and your back straight.
- Keep your head held high, your chin firmly forward, your shoulders back, chest out and stomach tucked in.
- Balance your weight evenly on both feet and keep your legs straight.
- If you have to stand for prolonged periods of time, then place one foot on a low stool and try to take regular breaks to sit down.

Driving

- Make sure that the seat is positioned close enough to the steering wheel so that the curve of your back is supported, that your knees are bent and either level with or higher than your hips and that your feet are able to reach the pedals, which should be squarely in front of your feet.
- Especially if you are driving long distances, use a small cushion, rolled-up towel or lumbar roll to support the small of your back.
- Ensure that your wing mirrors and rear-view mirror are correctly positioned to avoid having to twist around.
- Stop and take regular breaks to stretch your legs and move around.

Lifting and handling

- Always stop and think before attempting to lift something and take into account whether the weight can be safely lifted and whether there is any equipment available to assist.
- Make sure that you have a firm footing before attempting the lift, with your feet apart and one leg slightly forward to maintain balance.
- If the object that you are trying to lift is below waist level, keep your back straight and bend at the knees and the hips. Never bend forward at the waist with your knees straight, but instead let your legs take the strain and tighten your stomach muscles as you rise smoothly into a standing position without twisting.
- Keep the load as close to your body as you can when either lifting or carrying and keep your arms bent.
- If the item is heavier at one end than the other, always keep the heavier end closest to you.

- Avoid lifting heavy items above waist level.

- When carrying an object, take small steps, move slowly and avoid any sudden movements.

- Always keep your head up and your eyes fixed ahead of you rather than on the load that you are carrying.

- Use your feet to turn your body to avoid twisting your back or leaning sideways.

- If you are carrying items in both hands, such as shopping bags or luggage, try to distribute the weight evenly on both sides of the body.

- When setting down an item or items that you have been lifting or carrying, make sure that your feet are apart and then bend at the knees and hips whilst tightening the stomach muscles and keeping the back straight.

Lying down and sleeping

- Choose a firm mattress or, if necessary, place a board under a softer mattress to provide support.

- Try to avoid sleeping on your stomach as this can cause strain on your back and neck, especially if the mattress is not firm.

- Ideally, your sleeping position should maintain the natural curves in your back. If you sleep on your back, try placing a pillow under your knees or a lumbar roll under the lower part of your back, and if you sleep on your side, then keep your legs slightly bent and place a pillow between your knees. Do not, however, sleep on your side with your knees pulled up to your chest.

- Support your head with a pillow which is just thick enough so that your head and neck are in a normal position rather than using thick pillows which force your head up at an angle. The pillow should only be under your head and not your shoulders.

- When rising from the bed, avoid bending forward at the waist, but instead turn on to your side, pull up your knees, swing your legs over the side of the bed and use your hands to push you into a sitting position.

The above are general guidelines which are suitable for the majority of people, but if these in any way contradict the specific advice given to you by your healthcare professional, then the latter's guidance should be followed. In either case, however, if you find that levels of pain are increasing or that pain spreads to other areas of the body, do not hesitate to seek your physician's advice.

Herbal medicine

As well as the numerous types of pharmaceutical drugs that are available for treating the pain and stiffness which typically accompany neck and back injuries and conditions, a variety of preparations made entirely from plant material has also proved to be beneficial for some people. As certain herbal preparations can be dangerous for certain groups of people and some react with pharmaceutical medications, however, it is important to seek the advice of your physician before using a herbal remedy for neck and back or any other type of pain or symptoms.

■ **Devil's claw** – devil's claw, so named because of the appearance of the plant's fruit, has been used for its medicinal properties in Africa and Europe for centuries and is probably one of the best-known natural preparations for treating pain and inflammation. It is available in a variety of forms including pills, powder and capsules and there is evidence that it has proved particularly useful in reducing pain and improving physical function in patients with osteoarthritis in particular. Those with neck and lower back pain originating from other conditions, however, also seem to respond equally well to this as to prescribed pharmaceutical anti-inflammatory medication and the plant has been found to be very useful in helping to alleviate joint, ligament and tendon problems. The two main active ingredients in devil's claw are harpagoside and beta sitosterol, which offer analgesic, anti-inflammatory, sedative and diuretic properties.

■ **Capsaicin cream** – capsaicin is the active ingredient in chilli peppers and is what causes the burning sensation that we feel when we eat spicy foods containing chilli peppers. For pain relief, it is sold over the counter in different strengths in the form of a cream which is rubbed on to the skin and it works by depleting substance P and interfering with the transmission of pain signals to the brain. The cream generally causes a warm, burning or stinging sensation wherever it touches and this may last throughout the first few weeks of use. Great care needs to be taken with its use, however, in order to avoid it being inadvertently introduced into the eyes or any other sensitive area of the body. The pain-relieving effects of capsaicin cream are only short-lived, so re-application at regular intervals is necessary to achieve optimum results. In the case of muscle, nerve and joint pain, the cream often works fairly quickly, but those suffering from arthritis have noted that it can take a week or two of regular application before it takes effect.

■ **White willow bark** – white willow bark is often known as the 'herbal aspirin' and indeed its active ingredient, salicin, was used in the development of aspirin back in the 1800s. Although white willow bark is believed to contain other components which have antiseptic, fever-reducing, antioxidant and immune-boosting properties, salicin is known for easing pain and reducing inflammation. Some studies have shown that it is equally as effective as aspirin, but at much lower doses, which is thought to be because of the other components in the bark. Many find it particularly useful in cases of lower back pain and osteoarthritis.

■ **St John's wort** – although most often known for its ability to relieve minor to moderate depression, seasonal affective disorder (SAD), obsessive-compulsive disorders and premenstrual syndrome, St John's wort also has anti-inflammatory properties which make it particularly useful for nerve pain and arthritis. Available in tablet and powder form, St John's wort can also be brewed as a tea, but care needs to be taken with its use as it does interact with a wide variety of other medications. Some people who use St John's wort experience side effects such as:

■ nausea;
■ dizziness;
■ headaches;
■ constipation;
■ dry mouth;
■ confusion;
■ tiredness;
■ hypersensitivity of the skin to sunlight.

■ **Lavender** – lavender is a hugely popular plant for alleviating lower back and neck pain and so comes in a variety of forms. Specially-made neck wraps and pillows, including those which are micro-waveable, can be found in the shops and online, and the oils which are derived from the flowers are also used to make aromatherapy and massage oils which many find provide a good level of pain relief.

■ **Arnica** – arnica is another one of nature's wonderdrugs containing pain-relieving and anti-inflammatory components which often works extremely well in cases of acute or chronic neck or back pain. Used in the form of a cream or a gel, it is extremely effective for strains, sprains, bruising and swelling, but also works equally well for many people suffering from joint pain or arthritis and for bone breaks and fractures. Arnica should never be used internally, or on open wounds or broken skin, and some find that when it is used over prolonged periods of time, it can result in skin irritations. It has also been found to aggravate eczema in some people.

■ **Menthol** – widely recognised as an ingredient of toothpaste and mouthwash, menthol is a powerful natural pain reliever which comes from the mint and peppermint plants. Not only does it produce a numbing effect when applied to the skin, but it also increases blood flow by widening the blood vessels so that essential nutrients and other medicinal ingredients contained in the preparation can be carried to the area, as well as tricking the brain into relieving the heat of inflammation. In addition to being available in the form of creams, lotions and gels, it is also impregnated into patches or plasters which can be applied directly to the skin. Often it is combined with camphor, which also acts as a pain reliever and helps to increase circulation, providing relief from both pain and stiffness.

■ **Kudzu** – kudzu has been used in China and Japan for centuries for a bewildering variety of purposes, from treating heart attacks to alcohol abuse. In relation to neck and back pain, however, it is its power to interrupt the body's inflammatory response and so reduce inflammation which makes it particularly useful. Normally taken in the form of capsules, it seems to affect the body in a similar way to the hormone oestrogen and is therefore contraindicated for those taking tamoxifen or using oral medications for diabetes.

12

The Role of Cognitive Behavioural Therapy

Although it would be convenient to think of managing pain simply by treating physical symptoms, as I explained at the very start of this book, the International Association for the Study of Pain describes pain as 'an unpleasant sensory and emotional experience … ', which clearly indicates a psychological component. That does not mean to say, of course, that those who experience chronic pain conditions necessarily suffer from psychological disorders, but simply that the way that we humans think affects how we feel. Hence the reason why those who accept serious or chronic conditions or illnesses and develop and retain a positive mental attitude experience lower level symptoms and reduced amounts of pain. Such people are also more likely to remain active and exercise regularly, which also contributes greatly to reducing the severity of their symptoms.

Suffering day in and day out from what might be severe levels of pain when there is no end in sight and even strong pharmaceutical drugs do not appear to be helping is a devastating experience which impacts at many different levels and can lead to patients getting stuck in a vicious circle. As pain causes them to restrict their activities, so stiffness and weakness progress and they are able to do even less. Their home, working and social lives are all affected and relationship and financial concerns and feelings of isolation and low self-esteem begin to arise, all of which cause stress which exacerbates pain and other symptoms. On top of this, pain medications may be causing unpleasant side effects which send sufferers into an ever-increasing downward spiral.

People experience pain differently, and two individuals who present with almost identical conditions at similar degrees of severity can react in entirely different ways. The reasons for this might relate to their age, their gender, their past experiences, levels of fear or stress and whether or not they are in a state of depression. If you think about it, even the way that our parents taught us to react to pain when we were children, either taking a more relaxed view or flying into a panic every time we fell and grazed a knee, can still affect us well into our adult lives and help to determine our levels of fear and so on. Treating just the physical symptoms of neck and back pain, therefore, without addressing the psychological factors underlying the injury or condition, in many cases does not go far enough and does not allow the patient to be restored to maximum levels of either mental or physical fitness or a good quality of life.

Cognitive behavioural therapy, or CBT as it is known for short, although it is a psychological treatment, is one which is commonly used as part of a comprehensive pain management programme for those who suffer from chronic pain conditions, as well as those with serious or even life-threatening illnesses such as cancer and AIDS. It works by altering the thinking (cognitive element) of the patient with a view to making beneficial changes to behaviour (behavioural element) and may take place on a one-to-one basis or as part of a group session. Rather than concentrating on exploring any deep-rooted or long-standing psychological problems as some other types of psychotherapy do though, when used in this arena, the aim of CBT is to help individuals to improve the way that they manage and cope with the pain which has resulted from their conditions or injuries. Not only is it therefore a highly practical form of treatment, but also one which teaches patients the tools for ensuring long-term recovery.

Cognitive behavioural therapy is very much centred around problem solving and so allows sufferers of chronic pain to take back the control of their own lives. As well as helping to identify patterns of negative thinking which contribute to emotional and thus physical distress and teaching patients how to replace these with more positive and productive ways of thinking, it also deals with:

- relaxation training;
- planning and pacing activities;
- stress management;
- anger management;
- developing effective challenges to bring about improvements in physical function.

The result is that most people who undergo CBT experience increases in their coping abilities and their levels of self-esteem, reductions in their levels of fear and their feelings of hopelessness, improvements in their mood and associated reductions in the severity of their physical symptoms.

Remember, even though CBT is a psychological treatment, if it is something which is recommended by your pain management specialist this does not mean that he or she considers you to be suffering from deep-rooted psychological issues. The treatment is carried out in the direct context of your neck or back condition and is aimed specifically at helping you to develop a new and improved approach to coping with it.

Part Four

The Medico-Legal Implications of
Neck and Back Problems

13

Personal Injury Claims and the Burden of Proof

Many of the conditions which cause neck and back pain are ones which occur as a natural result of the body's aging process or because of infections, diseases or developmental disorders. In other cases, however, damage to the spine is incurred due to accident or injury, which the sufferer may or may not have been personally responsible for.

One of the major causes of neck and back injuries in today's society is motoring accidents, with whiplash claiming by far the greatest number of victims. Because this type of injury is most often sustained when a vehicle is 'rear-ended', rather than the injured driver or passenger being held legally responsible for the collision, it is the driver of the vehicle which failed to stop in time who is considered to be at fault. In cases such as these, therefore, the injured party has a legal right to pursue compensation from the driver of the other vehicle in relation to any medical fees or loss of earnings which may have resulted from the accident, as well as for the pain and suffering that he or she has experienced.

Of course, motoring accidents are not the only kind in which someone else might be considered to be liable. Accidents at work which happen as the result of an employer's negligence, such as the failure to provide necessary tools and equipment or the training required to do the job properly are other examples of those which could potentially lead to an individual pursuing a personal injury claim. Trips, slips and falls which occur because of spillages on shop floors or inadequate warning signs or because local authorities have failed to ensure that pavements have been properly maintained can also be grounds for pursuing a claim.

Quite often, those who suffer from neck or back pain as the result of somebody else's negligence fail to make a personal injury claim, and one of the most common reasons for this is because the symptoms of their injury do not manifest themselves until long after the incident took place. Generally speaking, however, claimants have a whole three years in which to initiate a claim and in cases where, for example, the nature of the injury took even longer than this to become apparent, it is sometimes possible for this deadline to be extended further.

Another reason why some prefer not to pursue personal injury claims, even though they may have suffered considerably as a result of someone else's negligence, is because of a lack of appreciation of how these work or a misconception that they will prove costly. Personal injury claims, however, are quite different from what are often expensive criminal cases, because the burden of proof is not the same. In a criminal law case, the lawyer for the prosecution is required to show 'beyond reasonable doubt' that the defendant is guilty if he or she is to win the case, and this of course means providing substantial amounts of detailed evidence which take a great deal of time and money to gather. In a personal injury claim which is dealt with under civil law, on the other hand, the burden of proof lies on the balance of probabilities. Hence, if the lawyer who is acting on behalf of the claimant can show that what his or her client says is, on balance, more likely than the claims made by the person who caused the accident, then this is sufficient for the personal injury claim to be accepted.

Clearly, anyone who is considering making a personal injury claim needs to be represented by a lawyer, whose job it is to prove that the other party was responsible for the accident and the consequential injuries, and to persuade the other side to pay out a sum of money which is commensurate with the extent of the victim's pain and suffering and fully compensates him or her for any related expenses. In order to do this, the lawyer needs to demonstrate that the neck or back pain from which his or her client is suffering occurred as a direct result of the other party's negligence, which requires the production of a qualified medical expert's report. This report is made available to the other party's legal representative who then has a specified amount of time to consider its contents and decide whether to accept or reject the claim. If he decides to accept, then an appropriate settlement is negotiated and agreed and, in most cases, the person pursuing the claim does not have to pay for any of the costs associated with the claim.

The medical reports which are provided in support of personal injury claims do, of course, vary in terms of their contents and format, but in order to be most effective, these should give a detailed account of your medical status. While some practitioners may only be qualified to speak to the physical aspects of your condition, one of the benefits of dealing with a multidisciplinary pain management facility is that the body of evidence is likely to be broader and able to take into account any emotional and psychological effects that you may have suffered, which in turn might impact on the level of compensation that you are ultimately awarded. Because a range of different experts is on hand to assess your condition using a variety of specialised techniques, this also means that the evidence put forward in the report is stronger.

To give you an idea of what a comprehensive medico-legal report might contain, those provided by the London Pain Clinic consist of:

1. Details
2. Content
3. Introduction
4. Methodology
5. History
6. Examination
7. Opinion
8. Prognosis
9. Medico-legal declaration
10. Curriculum Vitae

Wherever possible, the reports that we produce will conclude with our recommendations for treatment.

Of course, no individual or company (it is normally an insurance company which is responsible for paying the compensation and footing the bill for the case costs) is going to pay out what might be a considerable sum of money by way of compensation unless they absolutely have to, however, which does mean that personal injury cases tend to be adversarial by nature. Unless the legal representative who is acting on behalf of the compensator considers it pointless to make any defence, he or she will also present evidence to support his or her rejection of the claim. Ensuring that you are represented by the strongest legal and medical experts, therefore, is absolutely vital in ensuring that your case is successful and that your claim is dealt with expediently.

14

Medico-Legal Experts and Personal Injury Solicitors

Pursuing a successful personal injury claim not only requires the expert knowledge of a solicitor who is experienced in dealing with such cases, but also a high degree of medical expertise in the area which pertains directly to the nature of the injuries sustained by the claimant. In order for the other party to be persuaded to accept the claim, the medical expert clearly needs to be able to demonstrate his or her specialist knowledge and outstanding reputation within the field, but where personal injury claims are concerned, this in itself is not enough. Just because a medical practitioner is highly trained and qualified and is an expert in assessing, diagnosing and treating patients, does not necessarily mean that he or she also has the skills or the experience to present medical evidence in such a way as to be totally convincing in a legal sense.

Medico-legal experts are highly-trained and qualified individuals who not only possess the knowledge and skills to make the kind of expert clinical assessment which is required for a personal injury case to be accepted and taken forward, but also the experience and abilities necessary to present his or her findings in such a way that the evidence appears irrefutable. As the name suggests, therefore, the role of such an expert is one which cuts across both the medical and legal disciplines, so ensuring the greatest chances of achieving the first aim, that of winning the case.

The reason why I say that winning a personal injury case is only the first objective is, of course, that even if the financial payout involves a substantial amount of money, this in itself can do nothing to affect the pain and suffering and the quality of life of the person who has sustained the injury. The most effective way to treat and manage injuries and conditions which cause neck and back pain is via a multi-disciplinary programme provided by a specialist. In addition to providing the best possible assessment and diagnosis required to win a personal injury claim, therefore, the right medico-legal expert is qualified to provide the highest quality standards of multi-disciplinary treatment to return the sufferer as close as possible to his or her former state of health.

Of course, the use of a medico-legal expert does not dispense with the need for a solicitor to represent your case, and once again the calibre of the legal representative that you choose will not only help you to win your personal injury claim, but something else too.

Although it might be easy to think of the process following an accident to be neatly and logically ordered (i.e. accident – claim – compensation – treatment), of course in reality it frequently does not work like this. You may, for instance, have paid out for medical fees in relation to diagnosis and treatment before appreciating the link between your symptoms and the earlier accident, in which case the order would be: accident – treatment – claim – compensation, a situation which would clearly see you out of pocket until your compensation was paid. Having decided to pursue a claim, however, something else that a strong legal representative, backed by an experienced medico-legal expert, may be able to do is to secure one or more interim payments on your behalf. Even if you have not yet invested in treatment but your injury has affected your earning capability, an interim payment could be used to improve your quality of life during the time that it takes for your claim to be fully settled.

The amount that your solicitor might be able to negotiate on your behalf for an interim payment will naturally depend on the expected final payout, but provided that it does not exceed what would be considered to be a 'reasonable proportion', there is every possibility that it will be accepted. If the case drags on or you need to incur further costs while the claim is in progress, such as for more treatments, then your solicitor can negotiate additional interim payments for you, with these being deducted from the agreed settlement figure when the case is concluded.

Many people are discouraged from pursuing a personal injury claim because of fears of enormous legal costs, especially since legal aid is not available for such claims. Many personal injury solicitors nowadays, however, work on a 'no win, no fee' basis, which means that only if your case is successful and you receive compensation for your injuries will you have to pay for your legal representation. If this is the case and you do win, normally you would not have to pay for court or medical report costs, as these are generally settled by the other side.

Obviously, if a solicitor is going to take on your case on a 'no win, no fee' basis, then he or she needs to be persuaded that the chances of success are high. By choosing an experienced medico-legal expert who specialises in cases of neck and back pain, you will be able to arm yourself with the strongest possible medical evidence to convince a solicitor to take your case on and, working hand in hand, the two will maximise your chances of securing higher levels of compensation on your behalf.

Conclusion

On any day of the week, millions of people all around the world will find themselves suffering from the effects of neck or back pain, and only relatively few individuals will make it through their lifetime without experiencing at least one painful episode. Although some will make a natural and speedy recovery, unfortunately many others will continue to suffer for months and even years into the future.

One of the greatest sadnesses with respect to neck and back pain is that so much of the physical, emotional and psychological suffering is unnecessary. All too often, patients are provided with little or no education regarding the nature of their complaints and are offered only a very limited choice of treatment options, some of which have only minimal effect or come with equally distressing side effects. In many cases, no attempt whatsoever is made by the medical profession to address anything other than the direct physical implications of the condition and so acute cases frequently develop into chronic cases and the lives of chronic sufferers are left to continue on a vicious downward spiral.

Human beings are complex creatures whose physical well-being is inextricably linked with their emotional and psychological health. Far from being just a physical sensation, pain is also an emotional experience which can literally drive us into despair and hopelessness, and so tackling it from all angles is essential if full and lasting recovery is to be achieved. Dealing with pain symptoms might improve levels of comfort, but it will do little or nothing on its own if mobility issues are not addressed and the sufferer is still unable to take part in work or social activities or continue with normal day-to-day life. If posture, stress or weight issues are not dealt with, then physical pain will merely be aggravated, and if depression and anxiety are not treated then the patient will not only continue to live a life full of fear and despair, but will also lack the motivation to help him or herself.

Continuing amounts of time and research go into understanding chronic pain conditions and the effects that these have on the lives of sufferers. Almost without exception, findings indicate that those who take part in multidisciplinary treatment programmes experience the most significant and beneficial effects and that those who approach their conditions with a positive attitude and a commitment to their own health and well-being live happier and more successful lives with less or no pain. Even if their conditions are incurable, these people feel able to take control of their lives and you too can do the same.

I sincerely hope that this book has helped to demystify some of the main causes of neck and back pain, as well as to provide a greater sense of awareness in terms of your treatment options and the ways in which you yourself can go about tackling some of the practical and emotional issues which you may find yourself faced with as a result of your condition. Neck and back pain may be common, but all too often people suffer alone and so I would urge you to reach out for whatever help you require. If you feel that there is any further information, advice or support that I can offer, then please do not hesitate to contact me. Remember, life is short and you deserve the very best that it has to offer!

With all best wishes,
Dr Christopher Jenner MB BS, FCRA
London Pain Clinic
www.londonpainclinic.com

Index